Aromatherapy and massage

for mother and baby

Aromatherapy and massage

for mother and baby

*How essential oils can
help you in pregnancy and
early motherhood*

Allison England

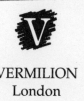

VERMILION
London

To my children

1 3 5 7 9 10 8 6 4 2

Text © Allison England 1993, 1999

Allison England has asserted her right to be identified as the author of this work under the Copyright Designs and Patents Act 1988.

First published in 1993 by Vermilion
This new edition published in 1999 by Vermilion
an imprint of Ebury Press
Random House, 20 Vauxhall Bridge Road, London SW1V 2SA

Random House Australia (Pty) Limited
20 Alfred Street, Milsons Point, Sydney, New South Wales 2061, Australia

Random House New Zealand Limited
18 Poland Road, Glenfield, Auckland 10, New Zealand

Random House South Africa (Pty) Limited
Endulini, 5A Jubilee Road, Parktown 2193, South Africa

The Random House Group Limited Reg. No. 954009

A CIP catalogue record for this book is available from the British Library.

Illustrations: Wendy Henry

ISBN 0 09 182275 0

Papers used by Vermilion are natural, recyclable products made from wood grown in sustainable forests.

Typeset by Digital Type, London
Printed and bound by Biddles of Guildford

Contents

Foreword   vi

Introduction   vii

Acknowledgements   viii

1 The benefits of aromatherapy in pregnancy   1

2 Aromatherapy and essential oils explained   8

3 A history of essential oils   15

4 How to use essential oils   21

5 A guide to essential oils   29

6 Pregnancy massage   42

7 Aromahelp for discomforts in pregnancy   50

8 Aromahelp for labour and birth   68

9 Postnatal care and adjusting to motherhood   79

10 Breast-feeding   86

11 Getting back into shape   90

12 Post-baby skin and hair   98

13 Baby massage   106

14 Aromahelp for baby problems   111

15 Preconceptual care   124

16 A reference guide to essential oils   127

Glossary of medical terms   144

Addresses   145

Index   148

Foreword

Aromatherapy is escalating in popularity and what a good thing too, as essential oils are, in my opinion, safe, non-toxic and extremely pleasant to use.

I am a midwife at a District General Hospital which has 2,500 deliveries annually. I mainly work on a ward for antenatal and postnatal women where we have essential oils available. In 1986, some of my colleagues introduced me to aromatherapy. They already used oils personally and suggested that I start using them in our holistic approach to individualised care. One of the great things about aromatherapy is watching my friends become converted. My husband – the greatest sceptic of all – now uses oils in his bath every Saturday to ease his rugby-injured muscles.

So, once confident about the value of oils and following a day workshop by an aromatherapist, in 1987 I introduced lavender oil into the ward environment. In 1988, a quality assurance survey showed that 84 per cent of the patients who had used essential oils had found them useful. Most women find relief and comfort from a long warm bath containing lavender oil. It eases pain of early labour, it cleanses and seems to help heal perineal wounds following childbirth. Lavender oil also balances moods in that most emotionally unstable of times.

We now make regular use of five different essential oils, giving individual tuition to new midwives who want to help patients use them. They are told how many drops to use and the dangers of side-effects if they are used inappropriately.

Once advised about the oils, patients too have access to them and may self-administer them, mainly into bath water. The oils are also used in massage, as compresses, or for inhalation by putting one drop on a tissue or pillow.

Until recently the value of aromatherapy was purely anecdotal. Now several people have started researching into essential oils, so in the future the medical profession will have to accept the claims made for them and hopefully will promote such a lovely alternative.

Ailsa Dale, Midwife
Hinchingbrooke Hospital, Huntingdon

Introduction

As a practising aromatherapist, I have enjoyed working with people of all ages and types, but over the last few years I have begun to take a particular interest in the health of women during and after pregnancy, probably fuelled by my own experiences as a mother of five children. Pregnancy is such a special time in a woman's life that she deserves to be taken care of while she is taking care of the baby.

I have seen the health of many pregnant women improve during the course of aromatherapy treatments, just as I've witnessed other women in good health remain on top form. Patients also look to me for reassurance, and I think that sometimes, like a mother, an aromatherapist often has to be a counsellor, a dietician, a nurse and a friend who is good at listening, all rolled into one.

This book has been written around the many questions I am asked by mothers-to-be and new mothers, with whom I've shared my love of essential oils. It was conceived because I felt that these women in particular needed to fully understand how to use these powerful aromatic oils to their very best advantage – and there are indeed many advantages.

But wonderful as they are, essential oils should be treated with respect. Just because they are a natural product from the plant world does not mean they can be used without thought and care. I'm sure you are familiar with what I call 'the grandmother touch' and the saying 'Just an extra spoonful, dear . . . a little more will do you the world of good'. This may be well intentioned, but should never be applied to the use of essential oils, where less often means more. Like all things in life, our bodies need balance. We thrive on vitamins and minerals, for example, and they are found naturally in our bodies. With the correct amount all is well, but too much of even a good thing can provoke a negative reaction. For this reason, whilst essential oils are an excellent choice for pregnant women and the very young, they need to be chosen and used with great care.

Aromatherapy has quite rightly gained tremendous popularity in recent years. The enthusiastic flair with which journalists have written about it in women's and other magazines has encouraged many readers to try the exotic oils. However, few people, even those keenly interested in complementary therapies, fully understand its origins and applications. In this book I would like to explain a little more about aromatherapy, in particular how it can help you through pregnancy and early motherhood.

As a prospective mother (or father), you have so much to look forward to. Aromatherapy can play a small part in making everything even better.

'The Lord hath created medicines
out of the earth, and he that is
wise will not abhor them.'

Ecclesiasticus, Chapter XXXVIII

Allison England

Acknowledgements

First and foremost I would like to thank Shealgh Doyle for all her support and encouragement – without her this book would never have got on to paper.

My grateful thanks for their help and time go to midwife Ailsa Dale, for her advice and for taking the time to write a foreword showing such enthusiasm for aromatherapy; Lola Borg for sorting out and editing the manuscript whilst having a baby (Francis) and moving house(!); and my clients, without whom there would have been no knowledge gained.

My special thanks and love go to my husband, Michael, for his loyal encouragement; and my children, Nick, Charlotte, Sophie, Ben and William, for the summer holidays over all too quickly, the goodies they kept me going with and all the many, many meals they shopped, cooked and washed up for without too much of a grumble!

1

The benefits
of aromatherapy
in pregnancy

In my aromatherapy practice I see many mothers-to-be and each approaches her pregnancy differently. Some are excited and positive in their outlook, feel well and strive to be in the very best of health. Others are apprehensive. They feel they are entering unknown territory and worry about every aspect of pregnancy and birth, from losing their figure to how they will cope with the new baby. Many worry that the relationship with their partner will change.

Some women are not in the peak of condition and find the myriad discomforts of pregnancy – particularly in the last few months – leave them physically or emotionally drained, especially if they already have a family to care for.

New mothers, of course, have their own problems. They can be tired from feeding or the constant activity that comes with a new baby, and maybe have to cope with the after-effects of a Caesarean birth or an episiotomy.

The wonderful thing about aromatherapy is that it has something to offer all these women.

Aromatherapy is an entirely individual treatment aimed at making each mother feel at her best. It can be used to help prevent or cope with any problems that can arise in pregnancy or early motherhood. Individual mothers can turn to aromatherapy for very different reasons and in each case it will be appropriate and beneficial. It can provide a nurturing, nourishing treatment which will enhance well-being and self-awareness and can help to relieve minor ailments should they arise.

Where aromatherapy helps most

Below I have listed some of the most important ways in which aromatherapy could help you to enjoy your pregnancy and your new baby.

- It can help to deal with stress.
- It will aid relaxation, help develop a more positive outlook and therefore help with the birth. A happy, relaxed mother is one who is more likely to cope well with labour and to relax and bond with her baby afterwards.
- It can help with tiredness, aches and pains and provide relief from all kinds of minor ailments in pregnancy.
- It can back up and complement what is learnt at relaxation and antenatal classes. Women who have had aromatherapy are more likely to benefit from the relaxation techniques they learn.
- It can help to prevent stretch marks by helping to keep the skin well nourished, and aid in helping the mother to feel good about herself during her pregnancy.
- Mothers-to-be who experience the benefits of aromatherapy are more likely to be in touch with their own bodies and their pregnancies and that can only be good for both mother and baby.
- The caring touch of a massage from either a qualified aromatherapist or from a partner is highly therapeutic. In my opinion, a woman who can appreciate the touch and care she receives whilst being massaged is more likely to bond better with her baby using her own tactile sense. This can only benefit the child.

After an aromatherapy massage a mother-to-be will often report a feeling of extreme peace and well-being and remark that her face has taken on a look of tranquillity. It can also help to remove the tensions from her life. Naturally, aromatherapy cannot remove the day-to-day problems that life throws at us, but someone who is relaxed can deal with them all the better. Of course the best way to receive an aromatherapy massage during pregnancy is from a qualified practitioner (see Appendix for how to find one in your area), but having a massage at home from your partner as well can only help.

Success stories

To give you a clearer idea of the benefits of aromatherapy in pregnancy, I have included these accounts of patients I have treated, either when pregnant or postnatally, in my aromatherapy practice over the years.

Camilla

Camilla came to see me when she was four months pregnant with her fourth child. She was tense and tired, said she wasn't sleeping well and had been told aromatherapy might help. At first her answers to my general questions about her health were brusque; eventually she broke down into sobs.

She had recently returned to full-time teaching after what she described as 'years at home' with her children who were now 13, 11 and six years old. She had been delighted with her job, knew it would be hard work to manage with a family, but felt they could all muddle through. But now she felt everything had gone wrong. Unlike her other pregnancies, this one was taking its toll on her. She was snappy and on edge, and felt she was sinking and couldn't cope with the exhausting demands of working all day, running a home and looking after her family. She was worried about how she would cope with the new baby, even with the help of a child minder. She didn't want to resign from her job as she felt she might not get another chance like it again, and as her husband was building up a new business after being made redundant, they could do with the extra money.

Camilla had always been a 'manager' and never liked to ask for help. Over a chat, she agreed to talk to her husband and explain to him how tired she was, and to lighten her load by getting friends to help out occasionally with her after-school commitments such as ferrying her daughter to ballet classes. She agreed to tell her GP she was feeling low, but I suggested that, for now, we should concentrate on making her feel better in herself, so that she could relax and sleep more soundly. Aromatherapy cannot wave a magic wand over problems, but I believed that if she felt less tired and was in a more positive frame of mind, then she would be in a better position to find some solutions to her problems.

Camilla loved the smell of the neroli oil I used to massage her, saying that the smell alone made her feel more cheerful. Although tense when I started her first massage, she was far more relaxed by the time I had finished and provisionally booked another appointment for me for the following week. The very next day I got a phone call from her. After her massage she had slept for the first time in weeks, and asked if I could see her, instead of in a week, in three days' time. She continued to come twice weekly for three weeks and then weekly for the rest of her pregnancy. She called it her 'hour of bliss'.

To back up her treatment, I mixed a relaxing bath oil with ylang-ylang, neroli and lavender. Her husband also used the bath oil and reported that it helped him to unwind at night ant sleep well. I also made up an oil with mandarin and lavender to use particularly as a body oil, for her back, legs and feet.

Physically Camilla remained very well for the rest of her pregnancy. The occasional leg ache was soothed by a foot massage by her husband or eldest son (albeit for a bit of extra pocket money). She still had her job and family to juggle, but because she was feeling better and coping well, she was now looking forward to the birth. She became much more relaxed about delegating chores to the rest of the family and putting her feet up in the evenings.

After a very short labour, during which her sister-in-law (who was Camilla's chosen birth partner) massaged her with lavender oil, Camilla gave birth to a beautiful baby girl.

Jane

Jane was a physiotherapist who was familiar with aromatherapy. She sometimes used essential oils at the end of her treatments to ease aches and pains. Her patients, she said, enjoyed the 'hands-on' approach of massage, especially as so many physiotherapy treatments seemed to be all machines. She had also been impressed by the pain-relieving qualities of the essential oils she had used on her patients. Now she was pregnant, she wanted, she said, to receive some tender loving care instead of giving it.

This was Jane's first pregnancy and she was feeling fit and well. During her initial consultation, I asked which essential oils she had used on her patients, particularly as the sort of ligament and joint conditions she worked with called for strong oils such as marjoram, juniper and rosemary, none of which should be used in pregnancy. She assured me that as soon as she knew she was pregnant she had switched to gentler oils – lavender, camomile and sometimes sandalwood – and always in a low dilution.

Jane intended to keep on working as long as possible. She kept really well throughout her pregnancy and really relaxed during her aromamassage each week. I used tangerine oil in a base of avocado and almond oil for her massage, and mixed up a bottle for her to use at home. This also helped to keep her skin supple and prevent stretch marks. She used this oil at night, but as she had to be out of the house quickly in the mornings, she hadn't time to let it 'sink in' before getting dressed, so I also made her up a creamy, non-sticky tangerine gel, which she could apply liberally before dressing.

Towards the end of the pregnancy she found, like many women on their feet all day, that her legs ached. For this I made her a gel with lavender and lemon. This is a wonderfully cooling recipe, which drains the throb from aching legs and feet.

Jane had known early in her pregnancy that her baby was to be born by Caesarean section. She now has a little boy, who regularly enjoys an aroma baby massage from his mum.

Jenny

I never met Jenny personally, but shortly before her due date she contacted me with a very definite list of requirements. She wanted a relaxing bath oil for labour (and also one for her husband!), a labour massage oil with jasmine and lavender and then a soothing bath oil for after the birth. Her friend, she explained, had 'had a baby with aromatherapy' and recommended it.

I duly sent off a package and a month later received a very sweet, newsy letter. She had had twin boys and had been determined to have a drug-free birth. She had found the lavender and ylang-ylang bath oil I sent really soothing and relaxing and, under the watchful eye of the midwife, had been allowed to stay in the bath for longer than she'd expected during the first stage of her labour. In fact, she said, the other midwives kept popping in to find out what the marvellous smell was. The jasmine and lavender massage oil had been wonderful during the second stage and she hadn't needed any extra pain relief, much to the surprise of the nurses. She had been disappointed, though, that monitors had been attached to her abdomen at the end of the first stage and throughout the rest of the delivery to check the babies' heartbeats. The first twin was born quickly with good, strong contractions. With the second, she had to have her legs in stirrups as he was lying awkwardly and there was a chance that forceps might be needed. Luckily, she said, they weren't and although she hadn't quite had the 'stand and deliver' type birth she had planned, she was very happy it was without drugs and overjoyed to be the proud mum of two beautiful boys.

She had had a few stitches, but had used the lavender and cypress bath oil I had sent and the nursing staff remarked how quickly she had healed. As for the bath oil for her husband – yes, she reported, he had had some relaxing nights' sleep before the birth, so he was fit and ready when the twins came home.

Mary

I was initially contacted by Mary's mother-in-law, who was staying with Mary for two weeks while her son was on a business trip abroad. Mary was four weeks post-delivery. Jamie's birth had been long and difficult and she just hadn't picked up afterwards. She was tired and run down from coping with the new baby, who wouldn't settled in the evenings, and a three-year-old daughter who wanted Mary's attention constantly and wouldn't go to bed at night. Mary's mother-in-law, who was of the generation to whom 'bedtime was bedtime' no matter what, felt that Mary was being too liberal with her daughter and 'making a rod for her own back'. All this was creating tension in the family.

So Mary came to see me, looking tired and washed out, with shadows under her eyes, dry skin and limp hair. She said she felt utterly seedy and joked that her husband would probably take one look at her and jump back on the nearest plane.

Mary had breast-fed for the first two weeks after the birth, but was supplementing with bottles as she was so tired and Jamie cried so much she felt she wasn't satisfying him. She would have preferred just to breast-feed. We talked a little about life at home. She had been upset that her husband had had to go away on business – even though she understood it was really necessary and he had delayed work to be at the birth – and felt she needed his support. Having his mother to stay was a strain. She was very kind and meant well, but had a much more rigid way of doing things, whereas Mary preferred to take each day as it came – not always the right approach, she admitted, and she felt this was why Alex, her daughter, was playing up.

I gave Mary a massage with geranium – a good balancing pick-me-up oil – in a base of peach nut kernel oil, which was good for her dry skin but mostly because she liked the sound of it. For the dry skin on her face I used rose oil in jojoba and she took a bottle of this to use at night. To help her relax, I suggested a soothing bath each night with essential oils of lavender and bergamot. I also suggested that she should try drinking fennel tea to help increase her milk supply and should take a rest during the day when the baby was sleeping, letting her mother-in-law amuse Alex in the afternoons instead of trying to do it herself. She had been keeping Alex with her all day, because she was worried her daughter might feel jealous of the baby, but admitted that even a small child can appreciate when her mother needs a little time alone and that a loving granny is just the person to take over on these occasions. With the help of a doll I keep especially for the purpose, I showed Mary how to give a baby massage, which would help her baby sleep if he had any colicky pain. She agreed to try it after his morning bath to see if he liked it, so I made up a camomile massage oil for this.

Mary came again the next week and looked much better. Jamie had been a little suspicious of the first massage, but the subsequent ones had done the trick and he was sleeping most evenings. He was more relaxed and so was Mary. Her mother-in-law had also taken Alex out most afternoons while Mary had a sleep and was more relaxed if Alex wouldn't go to bed easily at night. Mary had stopped bottle-feeding Jamie completely and was breast-feeding frequently.

2

Aromatherapy and essential oils explained

What is aromatherapy?

The word aromatherapy means 'treatment using scents' and that is exactly what it is. Aromatherapy is a therapeutic and complementary treatment that reaches the very core of our senses through touch and smell, using the scents from aromatic oils to heal and uplift the body and spirit and make us feel better mentally and physically.

Contrary to popular belief, aromatherapy is not just massage with scented oils. Aromatherapists do use massage as an important and very valuable part of many treatments, but they also use oils in other ways – for aromatic baths and in creams, lotions, compresses and vaporisers.

Essential oils

Essential oils are the highly concentrated and potent oils which are used in aromatherapy. They are extracted or distilled from various parts of plants and trees, where they can be found in special secretory glands or cells. Some plants contain essential oils in their leaves or roots, others in their flowers, fruit, stem, bark or seeds. Oil of rose, for example, is found in the flower.

Extracting essential oils

Just to run through the names of some essential oils gives an idea of the diversity of their origins. Some, such as lavender, rosemary and marjoram, conjure up visions of an English country garden.

Others such as ylang-ylang or sandalwood suggest their more exotic origins.

With essential oils, like wine, there are good years and bad years, and like any other crop, their quality reflects that of the soil. The same oil may be weaker in therapeutic terms if extracted from a plant grown in poor soil. Some crops are harvested during the summer, such as lavender, whilst the flowers used to make essential oil of jasmine are gathered at night when their perfume is more pronounced. It takes many thousands of petals to produce floral oils such as jasmine and rose, as their secretory yield is not high. This is reflected in the price of these oils (they are among the most expensive). Other oils, such as tea-tree and eucalyptus, both with a medicinal and fresh smell, are more easily produced in larger amounts from a distillation of the leaves or sometimes the stems of their plants. These are therefore less expensive oils.

The most common method of obtaining essential oils from plants is by *steam distillation*. Plant matter is placed in a still. Steam is passed through, carrying oil particles from the plant matter into another container. Here the steam is cooled and returned to a liquid – now a mixture of water and particles of essential oils from the plant matter. The water separates from the essential oil, which, being lighter, floats on top and is then collected. This is the most suitable method of distillation for extracting aromatherapy oils and, in fact, purists believe that only an oil obtained in this way can be called an essential oil.

But there are other methods of extracting essential oils. With *solvent extraction*, for example, heated solvents remove oil from the plant material, leaving an odour-laden substance known as 'floral concrete'. This method is used for delicate flowers and resins and is more suitable for perfumery than aromatherapy oils. *Enfleurage* is also used for delicate flowers. This is a very slow process which involves flower petals being laid on glass frames smeared with grease. It takes up to three days for all the oil in the petals to be absorbed by the grease. Withered petals are then replaced by fresh ones. This process is repeated many times until the grease is completely saturated with flower oil. It is then washed in alcohol to extract this oil. *Expression* is a method used for citrus oils. In the past, the oils were squeezed out by hand and collected on sponges. Now this laborious task is performed by machines.

Some general properties and uses

If you imagine that they are rather like, say, the vanilla essence that is used in cooking, that will give some idea of their qualities, but obviously essential oils are much stronger, purer and more powerful. Although they are called oils, they are not oily like cooking oil and won't leave a greasy mark on paper or fabric. Their consistency is usually more like that of an alcohol, although some, such as myrrh or benzoin, are thick like runny honey.

Rather in the same way that each of the plants they derive from has its own flavour and personality, all essential oils have their own individual character or 'blueprint', an absolutely unique identity. Each has an ingredient list that reads rather like a laboratory report. Using only the sun's energy, plus soil, air and water, what evolves is a perfectly balanced cocktail of complex chemicals. It is this combination that gives each one its individual perfume along with its particular beneficial and healing properties. To date, it is impossible to produce an essential oil in its exact form synthetically. They are so potent they need only be used in tiny quantities – usually by the drop – to be beneficial and effective.

Essential oils have long been known to contain positive healing, therapeutic and cosmetic properties. Of this there is no doubt. Their use dates back as far as ancient Egypt and they are widely used today by the pharmaceutical and food industries. Peppermint is frequently used in toothpaste, for example, and petitgrain in many eau-de-Colognes.

Essential oils are natural antiseptics, some more powerful than others. It has been shown that they can kill airborne viruses, bacteria and fungi and can neutralise the germs that cause body odours. Unlike some synthetic topical preparations, they can help to kill germs without harming body tissue, when used correctly in dilution.

Some oils, such as camomile, are analgesic or anti-inflammatory and help to reduce aches, pain and swellings. Others, such as bergamot, have anti-depressant qualities and can help to alleviate insomnia, anxiety and mental or physical fatigue. Some oils have a great diversity of properties and uses. Oils such as lavender and tea-tree are powerful antiseptics with soothing and healing properties. Applied to a wound either oil would do a good job as an antiseptic, but tea-tree also has excellent anti-fungal properties and so can help conditions such as athlete's foot and thrush. Lavender, when diluted in a carrier oil and massaged into the skin, can help to relieve labour pains or soothe a headache. It can also help to disinfect a bucket of nappies when a few drops are added to a pre-wash soak. For those new to essential oils lavender should be their first choice as it has so many different uses.

When using essential oils at home, especially in pregnancy and on the very young, it is important to know which properties an oil has and whether it is, for example, sedating, antiseptic, stimulating or relaxing.

All oils, as I've said, have their own properties. But when two or more are mixed, another completely individual oil is made and the therapeutic effect or smell can be enhanced. This allows us to treat individual needs or conditions. It has also meant that most professional aromatherapists develop their very own 'time-tested' recipes. Some of mine are included in this book.

How essential oils get into the skin

'How can the oil from a fruit or a flower work its way into my body and make me feel good or soothe my pain?' This is one of the most common questions I am asked by my patients. In fact, aromatherapy oils work in two very distinct and different ways:

- by the sense of smell, and
- by absorption through the skin.

The sense of smell

The sense of smell is often taken for granted, but the human body is capable of registering and recognising thousands of different smells. Everything has its own individual smell. Your home, however clean and fresh it may seem to you, will have a recognisable smell to outsiders. How often have you heard people use the phrase, 'It doesn't smell like home'?

But there are certain smells that we have almost forgotten to recognise. All animals, including humans, produce odoriferous scents called pheromones. Animals have a far more pronounced use of these scents, employing them to warn one another of danger (hence the expression 'the smell of fear'), to attract one another sexually and to mark their territory, as anyone with more than one cat will known. They also use them to identify their own, which is why farmers will skin a dead lamb and use this to cover an orphaned one. The mother of the dead lamb, recognising the smell of her offspring, will then accept this new 'baby' as one of her own.

Humans smell too and not only with what we know as 'body odour'. Each person has a subtle and individual smell. Your dog will know you by your own odour and, likewise, a human baby within a few weeks of life will learn to recognise the smell of its mother (this includes babies that are bottle-fed) and prefer her company. Men and women too are responsive to one another's individual scents. Blondes, brunettes and redheads apparently all smell very differently. The preference of some men for blondes is put down to the fact that blondes are believed to exude a smell similar to babies (small children and babies smell naturally sweet).

Our pheromones changes throughout life, influenced by factors such as pregnancy, the pill, hormonal changes and illness. Diabetics, for example, can exude a smell like acetone and pneumonia has a dank smell. Babies and children smell differently from adults. From puberty a male could be described as 'musky', a scent which women in particular are supposed to find sexually appealing, which is why the musky scent exuded by the male civet cat (now thankfully synthesised) is incorporated into so many male toiletries such as aftershave.

A woman's pheromones change with her menstrual cycle, becoming sweeter around ovulation. Her own sense of smell is more pronounced then too (no doubt to seek out a 'musky' male). Males apparently also find women more attractive at this time. It is of course ironic that we spend a fortune on perfumes and deodorants, applying them liberally before a romantic evening, when the naked, natural smell we possess is more likely to get results. Women who live together have a tendency to begin to menstruate at the same time each month and this is attributed to natural scent regulation, when some subtle glandular odour is picked up. But perhaps the most astonishing example of how overlooked the sense of smell can be is shown by recent research into the impressive success of women at trout and salmon fishing (three records established in the 1920s by women anglers have still not been beaten). The theory is that the salmon, who can pick up waterborne chemical messages to a very great degree, are attracted by female pheromones. Apparently the odour of a man's hand can alarm or repel the salmon, whereas those of a woman will not.

On a less basic level, what all of this means is that smells can trigger both psychological and physiological responses in the body. Aromatic substances, such as essential oils, send out odour molecules. When we breathe these in, receptor cells high in the nose transmit impulses about the odour straight to the olfactory area of the brain. This area is closely linked to other systems that control the memory, emotions, hormones, sexual feelings and heart rate. The impulses work quickly, triggering neurochemicals that can be stimulating, sedating, relaxing or euphoric, and bringing about changes that can be both psychological and physiological.

This is why the sense of smell has such a powerful and immediate effect on the body and why aromatherapy can be so effective, especially in situations where the heart rate and respiration are affected by fear or anxiety, as in labour. It is hardly surprising that among the essential oils most beneficial for helping stress, anxiety and depression, are the lovely-smelling flower oils such as rose, neroli (from orange blossom), jasmine and lavender.

In theory, we are subject to a type of aromatherapy every day, any time a smell triggers off a response in the brain. If we unexpectedly catch a hint of a perfume associated with someone we love, for example, it provokes a pleasant, nostalgic feeling. Conversely, if we smell something we dislike, such as carbolic soap or damp roller towels, it can instantly transport us back to our schooldays. In *Remembrance of Things Past*, it is just the aroma of a madeleine cake that takes Proust back to his childhood. Smells can alert us to danger (the smell of smoke or something burning), warn us off certain actions (food or milk that has gone off informs us not to eat it), stimulate digestion and even make us more alert. The Japanese have done trials showing that lemon oil vaporised into the air can increase efficiency. All of which proves just how powerful the sense of smell can be.

The skin

The skin is the body's largest organ. It could be described as the packaging that keeps us warm, stops rain from getting in and stops our insides from falling out. But it is a lot more than simple 'wrapping paper'. It acts as an outer warning system, relaying messages to the brain about our environment by means of temperature, pain, touch, etc., and reflects the inner body by showing age and state of health.

Some people find it hard to believe that our skin is anything other than thick waterproof covering. To a certain extent this is true. We don't absorb bath water, for example. Neither do we absorb heavy, thick mineral oils, such as petroleum jelly which just leaves a greasy layer on the skin. But it is possible for the skin to allow through certain substances, if their molecular structure is small enough.

The skin is one of the body's organs of elimination. We lose sweat and other soluble wastes through the skin and so in the same way we can let things out, we can also let things in. Doctors are now increasingly administering medications, such as anti-angina drugs and hormone replacement therapy (HRT), by applying them to the skin, which means they bypass the digestive system and, in turn, are kinder to the body's internal organs.

Whether applied to the skin in a carrier oil or used in the bath, the tiny molecular structure of an essential oil enables it to pass through the skin. It travels via the hair follicles, diffusing into the blood stream, or is taken into the lymphatic and extra-cellular fluids. It is here at cellular level that the organic, therapeutic ingredients of the essential oil are broken down and are used by the body for the intended purpose, such as, for example, when you have massaged on camomile oil for its pain-relieving properties.

It can take anything from 20 minutes to seven hours for oils applied to the skin to be fully absorbed into the body, the time taken varying according to the amount of body fat (the more there is, the longer it takes), which is why aromatherapists request clients not to shower or bathe for at least seven hours after a treatment to ensure none of the oil applied is washed off.

After performing their healing functions on the body, essential oils are eliminated along with all the other body's wastes, such as sweat and urine, but leaving the body all the better for having been there and without any of the side-effects modern drugs can inflict.

3
A history of essential oils

'The way to health is to have an aromatic
bath and a scented massage every day.'

Hippocrates

'A woman lies relaxing whilst skilled hands rub warm, scented
oils rhythmically over her body ...' This description of a woman
of the 1990s enjoying a massage could apply equally well to an
Egyptian woman of around 3,000 years B.C. Although aromatherapy may seem like a relatively new branch of complementary
medicine, the practice of using oils for perfuming, healing and
religious ceremonies can be traced back thousands of years.

In the 1920s, when archaeologists uncovered the tombs of the
Pharaohs, they discovered jars of fragrant oils, still with a faint
aroma even after thousands of years. Egyptian mummies were
found to be so well preserved because the resins and essential oils
used for embalmment contained anti-bacterial and antiseptic
properties that prevented putrefaction and decay. Essential oils of
cedarwood, myrrh, galbanum clove and nutmeg were impregnated in bandages wrapped around the mummies.

In ancient Egypt, it was the priests who prescribed medicines and
who knew the power of oils, which they also used to alter moods in
religious ceremonies. Oils used were most likely not distilled (see
Chapter 2, page 9) but produced either by dropping aromatic plants
or resin gums into animal fat which was then left in the sun until
impregnated by the scent, or by steeping the plant materials in olive
or sesame oil. The basic method of distilling oils from plants that we
use today with essential oils, was reputed to have been discovered
by an Arab physician, Avicenna, in the tenth century.

There are frequent references to essential oils in the Bible. In
Exodus 20:26, for example, Moses in instructed by God to take
fine spices of liquid myrrh, fragrant cinnamon, cane, cassia and
olive oil and blend them into a sacred anointing oil. In the Book of

Esther, virgins especially chosen for the harem 'had to complete 12 months of beauty treatments specially prescribed for the women, six months with oil of myrrh and six with perfumes and cosmetics' before being taken to the king.

The infamous Cleopatra apparently knew of the aphrodisiac charms of oils and seduced Antony after bathing in jasmine with her room scattered with rose petals. Along with so much else of their culture, the Egyptians passed their knowledge and love of aromatic perfumes to the Greeks, who in turn advanced this by looking at the medicinal values of plants, perfecting the art of steeping flower petals in carrier oils, such as olive oil, for medicinal and cosmetic use.

During this period of history, Greek physicians, such as Hippocrates, Galen and Dioscoridese, were to leave their mark on the world through their writing and research into plants. Many of their findings have been confirmed by modern research in this century. Hippocrates (now known as the father of medicine, whose name is given to the oath doctors take today) was the first physician to observe how the course of an illness progressed and to use that knowledge when treating the next case he encountered. He was aware of the anti-bacterial properties of certain plants and once, during a plague in Athens, implored the populace to burn these plants in the streets so that the aromatic fumes could protect them.

Galen, physician to the gladiators, discovered he could mix vegetable oil with beeswax and water to produce a cream that was soothing and kept the skin soft. He had, in fact, made the first ever 'cold cream'. Greek soldiers, when going into battle, probably carried the first-ever 'first-aid kit' – a small bag containing myrrh, which helped to heal their wounds. Myrrh is still used for the same purpose today. I find it excellent for treating stubborn leg ulcers.

At the height of the Roman Empire, great emphasis was put upon the benefits of bathing. The rich and fashionable would have magnificent bathing areas built into their homes, large enough to hold parties, and would indulge in great long rituals of soaking in warm water. They used oils such as lavender (its botanical name, *Lavandula officinalis* comes from the Latin verb *lavare*, to wash) to perfume the water and followed these luxurious baths with massages, again using scented oils. They also carried out what we know today as a very efficient way of removing dirt and dead skin cells. A mixture of pumice and olive oil was rubbed all over the body, then scraped off with a narrow scraper called a 'strigil', leaving the skin soft and clean. Lesser mortals would, of course, attend public baths.

While Rome bathed, its armies marched and with them carried herbs and oils for medicinal and culinary needs. Where they invaded, they planted seeds. Many of what we regard today as typical English garden herbs, such as lavender, lovage, parsley and fennel, are a legacy from the Romans.

After the fall of the Roman Empire, teachings and books written on aromatics reached the Arab world. It was here that essential oil of rose was first distilled and with it came rose water, which is widely used even now in Middle Eastern countries, especially in cooking. Trade routes now flourished between East and West, bringing to Europe spices and aromatics from the East, including sandalwood from India. The perfumes of Arabia became much sought-after. Whilst the Romans had taken many herb seeds for foreign countries, the Crusaders took back to their own lands exotic perfumes and essential oils, with the knowledge of how to distil them. The essential oil trade had truly begun.

During the Middle Ages, the use of herbs and aromatic oils was commonplace. Cooking was performed with liberal amounts of herbs and spices, not only to enhance flavour, but to mask the taste of putrid meat. There was also widespread knowledge of the medicinal and antiseptic properties of plants.

In the larger, wealthier homes, there would have been a still room – a place especially set aside for working with herbs and plants (which must have been a joy to work in). It was here that all kinds of aromatic recipes would be made, including ointments, strong herbal waters and basic medicinal potions. Cloth sachets filled with dry herbs would be made to lay among linen and clothes as protection against moths. Mattresses and pillows, too, would be stuffed with sweet-smelling herbs and flowers.

Plants such as lavender, hyssop, thyme and mint were strewn on floors to help disguise the strong smells that came from no sanitation and lack of personal hygiene. Powerful herbs such as thyme and rosemary were hung in bunches around the house or burnt on the fire when illness threatened, as the inhabitants quickly learnt that wherever strong scents linger, illness is less likely to rear its head. The Middle Ages are now notorious for the unsanitary conditions in which the average person lived. Aromatic oils were used not just for pleasure and cleanliness – often they were the only means available to wage war on disease and pain.

During the late sixteenth and early seventeenth centuries, many herbal texts were written by physicians and apothecaries, such as Nicholas Culpepper, John Gerard and John Parkinson. These praised and detailed herbal remedies and catalogued strange new plants that were beginning to arrive from the New World. The trades of apothecary and perfumer flourished and it is interesting to note that in times of epidemics and plagues, it was people from these professions, working on a daily basis with essential oils, who frequently escaped illness.

By the 1880s, chemists were discovering how to synthesise quick and cheap equivalents to many healing herbs and other plants. Thus the modern pharmaceutical industry was born and as medical science advanced, herbal medicine was viewed with an increasingly suspicious eye. Although doctors used essential oils until the latter part of the nineteenth century as a routine part of the medicine kit, interest in them for general medical use began to fade. They became relegated to a lesser use in flavourings and for the perfume industry.

However, research into the properties of essential oils did continue. The first documented laboratory research into their antiseptic properties was carried out in Paris in 1887 by a Dr Chamberland. He confirmed (as did others after him) that essential oils can kill airborne viruses, bacteria and fungi where sprayed into the air. Sadly, in spite of this important information, the doctors and chemists of the day preferred the new synthetic types of medicine.

By the beginning of the twentieth century, essential oils, even though they had proved their worth countless times in practical use over the centuries, were confined to being pushed back on to laboratory shelves. However, it was in a laboratory that interest in essential oils was re-awakened, by a French chemist, René Gattefosse. His original interest in essential oils began purely by chance. During an experiment in his laboratory, he burnt his hand badly and plunged it into the nearest liquid. This liquid happened to be lavender oil and the outcome was that his burnt hand rapidly became less inflamed and painless and the subsequent rate of healing was extraordinarily fast. This prompted Gattefosse to spend much time researching into essential oils and their medicinal application, particularly in dermatology. In 1937 he published a book which he called *aromatherapy* – a name that would open up a whole new era for essential oils.

Inspired by Gattefosse's research papers, a French army doctor, John Valnet, began his own clinical research, using essential oils as antiseptics on soldiers he treated in the Indo-China war. He was so impressed by the results that he went on to treat war veterans with psychological problems using essential oils. He has since written many books and articles on aromatherapy, including *The Practice of Aromatherapy* which is now a standard text for every professional aromatherapist.

But the practice of aromatherapy as we know it today – combining essential oils with massage for health, beauty and well-being – was started by an Austrian biochemist, Marguerite Maury. Her husband was a homeopathic doctor and both of them took a great interest in all forms of alternative medicine. Based on her knowledge of essential oils, she undertook a programme of research, demonstrating just how effective they are when absorbed through the skin. She was particularly interested in their healing and rejuvenating properties. In 1962 and again in 1967 she received major awards for her work. As well as lecturing on and sharing her knowledge of essential oils, she opened several clinics in Europe, including one in London. In 1961 she published a book, *Le Capital 'Jeunesse'*, which has now been reprinted and is currently available in English as *The Secret of Life and Youth* (C. W. Daniel Company Ltd, 1989).

The history of essential oils in childbirth

In the Western world, the use of plant oils in childbirth, just as in general medicine, has come full circle. Until the middle of the nineteenth century, women usually gave birth with other women helping them, most likely women from their own family who had children themselves, or local women experienced in labour who had witnessed many deliveries. Normally men were only called upon for their powers of strength, to help 'pull a child out' from a mother weak after a long labour. Often this was at the expense of both mother and baby, unless it was a shepherd used to birthing difficult lambs, in which case the mother stood more chance of survival!

There were no drugs to ease labour pains, so these early midwives used the only things they knew could help – aromatic plants and other substances. Recipes and knowledge to heal and deaden pain were handed down from mother to daughter, along with panaceas for many other ailments. One of the substances used in childbirth was ergot, a cereal fungus that helps the uterus to contract. A derivative, ergometrine, is still used today in the injection given immediately after birth to help the uterus to contract and expel the placenta.

The Church disagreed with women being relieved of the pain of childbirth. According to the Bible, women were supposed to 'bring forth children in sorrow'. During the Middle Ages these

Church views, along with the politics of the day, often led to women with valuable knowledge of the pain-relieving power of aromatics and herbal remedies being associated with witchcraft.

Medicine advanced with the discovery of 'laughing gas' in 1772. The use of remedies administered by women faded as the use of drugs increased. In childbirth, substances such as chloroform and morphine were used along with scopolamine (known as 'twilight sleep' as it rendered the mother near-unconscious). Men were the authority on drugs – and with it childbirth – whilst midwives were considered second-class. Women became conditioned to the idea that birth meant pain and fear and that labour represented giving birth flat on their backs (not for any medical reason but purely for the convenience of the male doctor) and, most likely, heavily sedated.

During the 1930s, it was this fear of childbirth that Dr Dick Grantly Read observed in his patients which led him and others, such as Fernand Lamaze, to realise that childbirth without conditioned fear was possible and that mothers could partake in and enjoy birth without huge interference from drugs. By the late 1940s, a new era had opened up for women, encouraging the use of breathing methods, relaxation and massage as aids to a pain-controlled labour. The revival of aromatherapy over the last decade has led to it too becoming a highly acceptable form of treatment. Women can be in control of their pain and emotions using the healing powers of aromatics, known for so many centuries. They also now, rightly, have a choice as to how to give birth, and even for those in favour of modern methods of pain relief, aromatherapy and massage can still play an important part in the their labour, as back-up to conventional treatment.

In many hospitals, nurses who have taken aromatherapy courses are now using essential oils and they are beginning to be used in labour wards. At the birth unit at St John's and St Elizabeth's Hospital, London, one midwife told me that 'aromatherapy is a way of life here'. It is one of their first choices for pain relief in labour, and is also used postnatally and for baby care. Essential oils are also used at the delivery suite and postnatal wards of Hinchingbrooke Hospital in Huntingdon, where midwives are happy for mothers-to-be to bring in their own essential oils for labour or to use their supply. At this hospital, there has recently been a trial study to test lavender oil versus conventional treatment for the relief of postnatal perineal pain. The results have yet to be published. At last, aromatherapy seems to be gaining the status it deserves for labour and childbirth.

4

How to use essential oils

Essential oils can be worked into the body in several different ways. Below are listed the safest and most common ways of using them. Recommended oils and recipes for the various methods are included in the relevant chapters.

Massage

Massage is helpful for relieving stress and tension, aiding relaxation, easing aching muscles and for general pain relief, as well as for improving skin tone and general well-being. In aromatherapy massage the essential oils are added to a carrier oil, such as almond or jojoba, before applying to the skin.

Body massage

● Pour a small amount of pre-prepared massage oil in the palms of the hands ($^1/_2$–1 teaspoonful will do a back and leg adequately, unless the person receiving the massage has very hairy or dry skin).
● Massage gently into the body. Always massage towards the heart. Don't massage near varicose veins (glide around them) or on hot, swollen joints or when a fever is present.

See Chapter 4 for full instructions on body massage and recipes for oils.

Foot massage

A foot massage is wonderful for relieving tension and to revive and re-energise a tired body. It's also bliss for swollen or aching feet.

● Spread a little pre-prepared oil all over one foot and around the ankle.

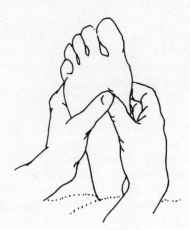

● With hands cupped around the foot and fingers steadying the front of the foot, use the thumbs to make circular pressures on the sole. Gently squeeze and press the foot as though you were trying to make it into a pliable piece of dough.
● Repeat with the other foot.

I guarantee that once you get the hang of it, those receiving the foot rub will beg for more.

Facial massage

A facial massage will help to care for any type of skin in every condition, both during and after pregnancy.

● Apply the pre-prepared oil very sparingly to the face and neck at night after cleansing.
● Always use gentle upward movements to apply the oil (to reverse the effects of gravity). Try not to drag the skin.
● If you are massaging someone's face, ask them to remove their contact lenses.

See Chapter 12 for full instructions and recipes for facial massage oils.

Aromatic baths

Aromatic baths are an important part of aromatherapy. Depending upon the oils used, they can be detoxifying, refreshing and reviving when taken in the morning, or sedating, calming and soothing when taken in the evening. They help to promote a restful night's sleep if taken just before bed and are helpful for reducing aches and pains.

For an aromatic bath during pregnancy:

• Add to a warm bath (never too hot), 2–4 drops of the chosen essential oil.
• Swish the water around to disperse the oil.
• Relax and soak in the bath for 10–15 minutes to enjoy the aroma and let the oils do their work.

Sitz bath or bidet

Both are used for washing and soothing the hips and genital area (particularly useful for just after childbirth). A sitz bath can be improvised by filling an ordinary bath with enough warm water to just cover the lower abdomen.

• Add to a sitz bath or bidet, 2 drops of the chosen essential oil.
• Mix the water well before stepping in.
• Soak for 5–10 minutes.

Children's baths

Children can benefit from aromatic baths as much as adults, but smaller quantities of oil should be used and even the mildest of essential oils must always be very well diluted. This is to avoid the child getting any drops of neat oil on his or her hands, which could then be rubbed into the eyes or mouth. Children also have very delicate skin that can be easily irritated.

The essential oils should be diluted in 10–20 mls (½–1 tablespoon) of full-fat milk. Goat's milk can be used if the child is allergic to cow's milk. Count out the drops (for quantities, see below) into a small bowl, add the milk, stir well and add to the bath water.

I recommend using no more than the following amounts of essential oil:

- For children of 5–12 years, add 2–4 drops of essential oil to the milk.
- For children of 2–5 years, add 1–2 drops of essential oil to the milk.
- For babies of over 3 months and very young children, add just one drop.

I don't recommend essential oils in the bath for babies under 3 months, and even then, they should not have them as a matter of course.

Footbaths

To a bowl of hot water:

- Add 2–3 drops of the chosen essential oil.
- Soak the feet for anything between 10–20 minutes.

Showers

Essential oils can also be used in a shower. The best way to use them is to wash as normal to begin with. Then add 2–3 drops of your chosen essential oil to a sponge or flannel and rub it all over the body while standing under the water and breathing in the vapours.

Compresses

Compresses are a wonder way to treat labour pain. They are also useful for any muscular aches and pains, sprains or bruises and to help reduce pain in general.

For acute inflammation, such as headache, swellings, sprains and wounds, etc., use a cold compress.

For chronic pain, such as backache, muscular pain, labour pain, earache, etc., use a hot compress.

For wounds or infected boils, the water should be previously boiled, and cotton wool or sterile gauze used as a compress.

- To 300 ml (½ pint) of water (either hot or cold according to which compress is needed), add 2–4 drops of essential oil.
- Agitate to mix the oils.

- Take a small cloth, flannel or towel and lay it on top of the water so that the oils are picked up on the underside.
- Lay this on the affected part. Cover with a small dry towel and leave in place until the cold compress has warmed to the body heat or the hot compress has lost heat.
- Renew as required.

Inhalations

Inhalations are used to clear the congestion that comes with colds and sinusitis. They can be extremely effective in unblocking the nose and helping to relieve the nasal passages.

Steam inhalations

- To a bowl of very hot (but not boiling) water, add 2–4 drops of the essential oil.
- Cover your head with a small dry towel (if you choose to), lean over the bowl and breathe in the vapour for about 1–5 minutes.

Steam inhalations are not suitable for asthmatics (they may of course use essential oils in the bath) or for children under ten years old. It is not safe for a small child to sit over a bowl of water. Children over ten years old should be attended at all times if they do have an inhalation and then only inhale the steam for a few minutes. In fact, it is better, if they have a cold, to sniff the oils on a tissue or have the oils vaporised in a room near them. Smaller children can have the same oils in the bath in a low dilution (i.e. 1–2 drops only). Or, for snuffly babies, the oils can be used in a special room vaporiser.

Using a tissue or handkerchief

To a tissue or clean handkerchief, add 1 drop of essential oil and sniff when required.

This is a very handy method of using essential oils if you have a cold, but it is also quite comforting postnatally if you can't have essential oils beside the bed in hospital. It's also very useful during labour.

To perfume rooms and purify the air

Essential oils can be used not only to add a delicious and relaxing aroma to a room, but also – depending upon the oil used, of course – to dispel bacteria or remove unwanted smells. There are many different ways of using essential oils to scent rooms:

With hot water

- To a bowl of hot water, add 2–6 drops of essential oil.
- Leave to stand in the room.

With a plant atomiser

- Fill a plant atomiser with 300 ml (1/2 pint) of water.
- Add 6 drops of essential oil.
- Then spray this mixture around the room.

With an appropriate essential oil, this is an idea way to dispel bacteria when there is illness in the house.

In a burner

A burner can be bought at most health food shops.

- Fill the top bowl of the burner with water.
- Add 2–3 drops of essential oil.
- Burn for as long as you choose – perhaps an hour – then extinguish the candle and allow the aroma to waft around the room.

Always ensure that the bowl of the burner is washed regularly to help stop the build-up of sticky, caramelised oils on the base.

On a lightbulb ring

Again, lightbulb rings are available at most health food shops.

- Follow the maker's instructions as to how to use them. Some are solid round rings and the oil can be dropped straight on to them; others have a reservoir inside, into which the oil can be dropped neat or added to water.

• Use 2–3 drops of essential oil and place the ring on to a lightbulb (in a table lamp is best). The heat from the bulb will warm the oil and send it into the room.

In a diffuser

Diffusers are available at major department stores and chemists. Follow the maker's instructions as to how to use them (they vary). When buying, ensure you purchase one with a bowl that is easily wiped clean, otherwise the diffuser will have a build-up of different essential oils on the base of the bowl.

On cotton-wool balls

• To a cotton-wool ball, add 2–6 drops of the chosen essential oil.
• Lodge behind the warm part of a radiator.

This method can be used in the rooms of babies or small children, but do take care and ensure the cotton-wool ball is placed where it cannot possibly be reached. If in doubt, don't use this method.

By scenting a fire

In wintertime it is wonderful to place just one drop of essential oil on to each log just *before* placing it on the fire. Remember, though, that essential oils are quite volatile and inflammable, so don't drop the oils straight into the fire. If you are lucky enough to have an Aga cooker, a couple of drops of essential oil can be dropped on to the back-plate to scent the room.

In a vacuum cleaner

This method can be used to freshen the whole house or remove fuggy smells.

• To a couple of cotton-wool balls, add 3–4 drops of essential oil.
• Pop these into the vacuum cleaner bag and they will refresh each room you vacuum. The aroma can linger for quite a time.

A word of caution

Essential oils are strong and need to be diluted before applying directly to the skin. They should always be used:

● in a carrier oil, or
● mixed with water, or
● added by the drop, to creams and lotions.

If not diluted, some oils, such as the citrus oils, could cause soreness and irritation. However, as in all things in life, there are exceptions to this rule. Two oils – lavender and tea-tree – can be used directly on the skin, but only in very small quantities – literally by the drop. Always use them either as directed by a qualified aromatherapist or follow recipe directions. Even so, some people with very sensitive skins may not be able to tolerate these two mild oils undiluted.

Essential oils should also never be swallowed or taken by mouth, as they are far too strong for the delicate lining of the alimentary tract.

Patch testing

If you have sensitive skin or suffer from eczema, dermatitis or any other allergies, such as hay fever, you may like to consult an aromatherapist before using any essential oils (see the Appendix for how the find one in your area). She may recommend, as I do, doing a patch test:

● To 10 ml (½ tablespoon) of carrier oil, add 2 drops of the essential oil you want to test.
● Smear a little on the inside of the elbow. There is no need to cover it. Leave the area unwashed for 24 hours.
● If any redness or itching occurs, do not use that oil as you may have an allergy to it.

If you are prone to allergies from nut or vegetable oils, you may also have to test the carrier oil and it is obviously better to do this before you test the essential oil. Follow the procedure as above by rubbing a smear of the carrier oil you wish to test on the inside of your elbow. Leave for 24 hours and if there is no reaction (such as redness or irritation) then proceed as above to test the essential oil. If there is an adverse reaction, try the procedure again with another carrier oil.

5
A guide to essential oils

There is a vast range of essential oils available now in the shops, but only certain ones should be used in pregnancy – those that are gentle and soothing. Stimulating oils should never be used as that effect is not particularly desirable in pregnancy (for a full list of oils to be avoided during pregnancy see pages 36–38). The following list of oils can be used safely.

Essential oils of greatest use during pregnancy

Lavender

(*Lavandula officinalis* – from the lavender flower)
Lavender oil is known as the 'great all-rounder', as it has so many uses. Anyone new to aromatherapy would do well to invest in some lavender oil. It is antibiotic, antiseptic and good for spots, grazes and minor burns. Used in skin creams, it can help cell renewal and minimise scarring. It soothes insect bites, fights off infections, relieves headaches and eases muscular aches and pains. In pregnancy, it is particularly useful for soothing aching backs, legs and ligament pain.

Another of the many qualities of lavender oil is its relaxing and anti-depressant properties. It has a mild sedative action so it helps insomnia and is a wonderful oil to use in the bath at the end of the day or to scent the room before sleep. It is, in fact, less an oil and more a medicine chest in a bottle and one of two oils (the other being tea-tree) that is gentle enough to be used – in small quantities – directly on the skin.

A smear of lavender oil applied to a minor burn is the perfect first-aid treatment, after plunging the burn into cold running water if possible. If this is repeated at intervals during the day, the lavender oil will help to remove the sting, stop any infection and minimise scarring.

Use for baths, massage, room fresheners and facial oils (see note on lavender oil under 'Essential Oil Safety' on page 36).

Mandarin

(*Citrus nobilis* – from the rind of the mandarin)
Mandarin has very similar properties to tangerine – calming, gentle and cheery – but has a slightly fresher smell. It is used in baths as its gentle tonic effects help to relieve fatigue. In leg and ankle massages, mandarin can ease fluid retention.

Use for baths, massage and room fresheners.

Neroli

(*Citrus aurantium* – from the flowers of the bitter orange tree)
An absolutely heavenly oil, neroli is also diabolically expensive but worth every penny as the aroma is so exquisite. It makes a wonderful face oil – good for dry or sensitive skin – and will help regenerate skin cells. It is one of the very best oils to use for nervous tension (I call it the 'anti-panic oil'), as it is so calming and relaxing. It is rumoured to have aphrodisiac qualities and is also a deeply peaceful oil. Neroli is excellent to use in pregnancy for its ability to promote healthy skin cells.

Use for baths, massage, room fresheners and facial oils.

Petitgrain

(*Citrus aurantium* – from the leaves and twigs of the bitter orange tree)
Petitgrain has similar properties to neroli – it is calming and soothing – but it is slightly less sedating with a fresher perfume, so it can be used as a cheaper alternative to neroli. It makes a lovely room scenter. It is particularly helpful in dealing with depression, either antenatally or postnatally.

A very special massage mix can be made using all three oils from the orange tree – petitgrain from the leaves and twigs, neroli from the flowers and orange from the fruit. Blended together they make what I call a 'total balance' oil, a very whole treatment, which I use for those who are depressed (see page 82 for recipe).

Use for baths, massage and room fresheners.

Tangerine

(*Citrus reticulata* – from the rind of the tangerine)
A nice happy oil and my favourite pregnancy oil, as it has a wonderfully uplifting smell. It helps to prevent stretch marks, which makes it excellent to use in massage. Tangerine is a beneficial oil to use when a tonic is needed as it is calming, gentle and good for the nerves and skin. As it is so mild, it is also a good oil to use for children or the elderly. Supposedly rich in Vitamin C, it is also well known as a tonic for upset stomachs.

Use in baths, massage and room fresheners.

Ylang-Ylang

(*Canaga odorata* – from the flowers of the tropical ylang-ylang tree)
This oil is very exotic and famed for its perfume. It has relaxing, restoring and aphrodisiac properties, and can even help to lower high blood pressure. It can also be used to help those who are tense and worried and is good used in a bath blend.

Use in baths, massage and room fresheners.

Essential oil for limited use during pregnancy

The following oils can also be used, but are not recommended in pregnancy as all-over massage oils. They are better added to gels and massage oils for specific areas, such as aching legs.

Cypress

(*Cupressus sempervirens* – from the evergreen tree)
Cypress oil has astringent qualities and is a gentle diuretic. I use it after the fifth month of pregnancy as it is particularly helpful, in a cooling lotion or gel, for varicose veins. Added to a bath, lotion or wash, it can help haemorrhoids (piles). Its gentle diuretic action can assist in decongesting fluid retention in heavy aching legs and swollen ankles.

Use after the fifth month of pregnancy, in local application gels, oils and washes.

Geranium

(*Pelargonium graveolens* – from the geranium plant)
This oil is known as an 'all-round balancer' as it puts the body
back into balance, but is quite a strong oil and best avoided as a
body massage in pregnancy. Geranium is astringent, refreshing
and relaxing and has a lovely aroma. In pregnancy I use it after
five months for the wonderful relief it gives to tired and aching
legs, as it is good for bad circulation.

Use in room fresheners and after the fifth month of pregnancy
in local massage gels, footbaths and oils.

Lemon

(*Citrus limonun* – from the rind of the lemon)
Lemon has a fresh, sharp citrus smell. It is refreshing, cooling,
antiseptic and aids the circulation. During pregnancy, it can be
used in a burner for morning sickness and in a local massage oil
or gel for varicose veins.

Use in local massage gels or oils, or as a room freshener.

Sandalwoood

(*Santalum album* – from the sandalwood tree)
Sandalwood is an exotic and relaxing oil, and an excellent facial
oil for dry or sensitive skin. In pregnancy it can be particularly
helpful for urinary infections.

Use in baths and for skin care.

Tea-Tree

(*Melaleuca alternifolia* – from the tropical tea-tree)
An incredibly useful essential oil, tea-tree is (along with lavender)
one of the essential oils mild enough to be used – in small
quantities – directly on the skin. This is usually to treat cuts and
wounds. It is an excellent anti-fungal oil, useful for cuts, spots and
wounds and as an inhalation for colds. For pregnancy, it can be
used to deal with thrush.

Use in local application washes and creams.

Carrier oils

All essential oils are blended and diluted into a carrier oil before using for massage. Only a very few drops of essential oil are needed in proportion to the carrier oil, rather in the same way that only a pinch of herbs or spices is needed in cooking. Carrier oils in aromatherapy are usually cold-pressed vegetable oils, rich in vitamins, proteins and minerals. They literally 'carry' the essential oil into the body and help lubricate the skin so the aromatherapist's hands can massage without dragging.

If you have very sensitive skin you may be allergic to certain carrier oils, so may need to try a patch test first (see page 28).

The following carriers oils are ones I have found most suitable for use in pregnancy, postnatally and for babies.

Sweet almond oil

(From almond nut kernels)
Rich in vitamins, this oil is particularly good for dry skin. It is light and easy to absorb and blends well with other oils. It can be used for face or body massage and is the most suitable oil to use for baby massage.

Use for face, body and babies.

Avocado

(From the avocado flesh)
Avocado is a very nourishing oil. It is usually mixed with other carrier oils as it tends to be a little too heavy to use alone, but penetrates easily and deeply and is therefore excellent for keeping skin supple and helping to prevent stretch marks. It is rich in protein and in Vitamins A, D and E.

Use for face and body.

Grapeseed Oil

(From the grape pip)
Grapeseed oil is popular for massage as it is light, non-sticky and usually doesn't provoke allergies. It is available widely – even in supermarkets – but it is best to buy a good-quality grapeseed oil, preferably in a glass bottle.

Use for face and body.

Jojoba

(Pronounced *ho-ho-ba* – from the beans of the shrub)
Jojoba is more of a wax than an oil, with healing and deeply moisturising properties. It penetrates the skin easily and, when used as a facial oil, jojoba mixes with and dissolves sebum and unclogs pores, which makes it an excellent oil to use on skin that is prone to acne.

It is also good for all skin types. It can be used by those with sensitive skin (particularly if the skin is also dry and wrinkly) and sparingly by those with eczema. It makes a good facial moisturiser – I use it as a base in all my facial massage oils – but is also excellent to use as a baby oil, especially where there is chapped skin.

Use for face, body and baby.

Wheatgerm Oil

(From the wheat 'germ' or grain)
Wheatgerm is a very heavy, strong-smelling oil, rich in Vitamin E, which is good for those with dry or lined skin. It is very helpful in preventing stretch marks and for healing scars left by spots, wounds or burns. One of nature's anti-oxidants, it will help to preserve and prolong the life of any blended mix of essential oils and carrier oils, such as a massage oil mix, if it makes up 10 per cent of the mix (i.e. in a 50 ml bottle, add 5 ml of wheatgerm to 45 ml of sweet almond oil).

It is not an oil I use, however, as it tends to have a fishy smell and must not be used by those with a wheat allergy.

Use for face and body.

Calendula

(*Calendula officinalis* – from macerated marigold flowers)
Calendula oil is very healing, has antiseptic properties and is good for inflamed or delicate skin.

I recommend using it in a cream for sore or cracked nipples and for babies, when it comprises 10 per cent of a mixture with sweet almond oil, to clean around any sore areas caused by nappy rash.

Aloe vera

(From the leaves of the plant)
Aloe vera is a gelatinous substances that is used frequently in creams and hair conditioners. It has moisturising properties and

can help to soothe burnt or irritated skin. When incorporated in a gel, aloe makes a good medium for adding essential oils to. They can be blended in either on their own or with other carrier oils. When buying aloe gel, ensure it contains a high percentage of aloe vera.

Use for face, body and baby.

Apricot kernel

(*Prunus armeniaca*)
A light textured and nourishing oil with virtually no odour, apricot is an ideal carrier medium for baby massage and for anyone who has, or is concerned about, nut allergies. It is suitable for delicate, sensitive and prematurely aged skins.

Use for face, body and baby.

Olive oil

(*Olea europa*)
Olive oil is heavy with a strong odour and a sticky feel. Although it is not recommended for an all-over-body massage, its soothing properties do have a beneficial action on dry, dehydrated and inflamed skins. Use it to nourish dry elbows, hands and heels.

Newborns frequently have dry peeling skin on their legs and feet. A little olive oil massaged gently into the skin can help to smooth any dry areas.

Use for face, body and baby.

Mixing the oils

As I've already said, because most essential oils are far too strong to use directly on the skin, they are diluted with carrier oils for massage. Often several different carriers oils are mixed together to form the base oil for a massage oil.

Mixing the base oil

The best base oil for a pregnancy massage is a blend of 80 per cent sweet almond oil and 20 per cent avocado oil:

• Take a clean, dry bottle.

- Pour in 40 ml (2 tablespoons) sweet almond oil and 10 ml (½ tablespoon) avocado oil.
- Mix well.

This base oil can be kept ready for use whenever you wish to mix an oil for massage by adding the desired essential oil.

Adding essential oils

As a general rule use only one drop of essential oil to every 4–5 ml (approximately ¼ tablespoon) of base oil. The quantities given below are the ideal ones to use for pregnancy massage oils:

- To 50 ml (2½ tablespoons) of base oil, add 10–12 drops of essential oil.
- To 100 ml (5 tablespoons) of base oil, add 20–25 drops of essential oil.

Don't be tempted to exceed the stated amount of essential oil, especially for oils to be used during pregnancy or for babies.

Some essential oils come out of the dropper very, very fast so, before making up your blend, practise with the dropper. This way the blend won't be spoilt.

Essential oil safety

Oils to avoid when pregnant

During pregnancy I always use, and advise clients to use, very limited amounts of essential oil. I have treated very many pregnant women and all of them have sailed happily and aromatically through their pregnancies. Nevertheless, as with all things taken in by or applied to the body during this time, you should be extra cautious, even to the point of being over-cautious.

So, in aromatherapy, we advise that certain essential oils should not be used in pregnancy. Some are considered too stimulating or too strong for a pregnant woman's vulnerable system and may cross the placental barrier. Others, known as emmenagogic oils, can stimulate menstruation. These should be avoided, particularly in early pregnancy. You may find some aromatherapists recommend not using these oils only during the first three to five months of pregnancy. I feel it is safer if they are avoided altogether. Enjoy the ones that you can use.

The only exceptions I would make to this rule are lavender, which although it has diuretic and emmenagogic properties, is so very, very mild that it can be used in early pregnancy, camomile (but both should be avoided if there has been any abnormal bleeding), and cypress, which I used in later pregnancy for local application to treat haemorrhoids.

I am often asked what effect using one of the oils that is not recommended would have on someone, say before they knew they were pregnant. Please don't panic if this has happened to you. The amount of oil used during, say, a massage is quite low. It is the continuous and indiscriminate use of these oils that we are concerned with. Just stop using any oils that are not recommended and inform your aromatherapist as soon as you even suspect you may be pregnant.

Before you buy any essential oils for pregnancy, familiarise yourself with the gentle ones suitable for pregnant women and do follow the recipes given in this book properly. Remember the quantities have been worked out very thoroughly and used in this way they are highly beneficial.

One last thing – I am frequently asked by patients if they can continue to use the herb form of essential oils that are not recommended. Essential oils are very much stronger and more concentrated than the herb or plant they derive from, so even if you are advised not to use certain essential oils, you can still use the herb. Oils such as basil, rosemary or mint should be avoided in pregnancy, but there is no harm whatsoever in using these herbs when cooking.

Oils to avoid when pregnant

Angelica	Hyssop	Peppermint
Aniseed	Jasmine	Rosemary
Basil	Juniper	Savory
Camphor	Lovage	Sage
Cedarwood	Melissa	Spanish Marjoram
Clary Sage	Myrrh	Sweet Marjoram
Clove	Marjoram	Tarragon
Cinnamon	Origanum	Thyme
Fennel	Parsley	

There seem to be so many oils available these days that there are bound to be some that I have not mentioned in this book. Don't buy an oil you have never heard of or read about, and if you have any doubts about an oil, leave well alone until you can find out full and reliable information about it.

Oils that should never be used in aromatherapy

Arnica	Jaborandi Leaf	Southernwood
Armoise	Mustard	Tansy
Baldo Leaf	Pennyroyal	Thuja
Bitter Almond	Rue	Wormwood
Calamus	Sassafras	Wintergreen
Horseradish	Savin	

A special word of caution

If you suffer from epilepsy or any sensitivity of the central nervous system, always consult an aromatherapist and let her advise you on your choice of essential oils. Some oils, if used indiscriminately or without care, could aggravate your condition or even trigger a fit. Do not use any of the following oils: fennel, hyssop, sage, wormwood and rosemary.

If you suffer from asthma, eczema, dermatitis or any other allergies, aromatherapy can certainly be of help, but ask the advice of an aromatherapist before buying essential oils. There may be some that you have a sensitivity to and she can advise you further.

Buying essential oils

Essential oils are the diluted essences from fruit, flowers and trees and it takes a great deal of work to produce even a tiny amount of essential oil. They are therefore expensive, but are incredibly potent and a little will go a very long way. They are usually sold in 10 ml bottles, which contain, on average, about 200 drops. As you can see from the recipes, 200 drops can go a very long way.

When buying oils, use the following guidelines. They will help you to find the best-quality oils, those with the highest therapeutic value:

● Always buy oils in dark glass bottles. Sunlight is the biggest enemy of essential oils and causes rapid deterioration. Always buy from shops with a high turnover, where the oils are not kept on a shelf exposed to sunlight.

● If you can, buy oils with a dropper insert already in the top of the bottle. This makes it much easier to measure out drops correctly. Always practise using the dropper before you make up a recipe as some droppers allow the oil out of the bottle at a much faster rate than others.

● Only buy small quantities of essential oils and blend as required with carrier oils.

● Never buy essential oils in plastic containers or decant them into plastic containers afterwards. Essential oils and plastic are not compatible. Some of the chemicals in plastics interact with the constituents in essential oils causing damage to the container or, at worst, spoiling the oil.

● When buying look for the phrase PURE ESSENTIAL OIL on the bottle. Only pure undiluted essential oils can be used effectively in aromatherapy. This applies as much for use in burners and baths as for massage. Any oil you buy that isn't pure essential oil may smell nice, but it won't have the same therapeutic effect as a pure oil. Similarly don't buy anything labelled AROMATHERAPY OIL, as the same applies.

● Buy the most expensive oils you can. Price is a good indication of quality. If you see a shelf of different oils that are all the same price, don't buy any of them. Neroli, for example, can be 20 times more expensive than lavender. Buy from a reputable source.

Storing essential oils

All essential oils will deteriorate unless stored correctly. If left unopened and stored in perfect condition they could probably keep for five years or more, but once opened they deteriorate rapidly. This is because once a bottle of essential oil has been opened, air gets inside the bottle. Each time the top is taken off more air travels inside and eventually causes oxidisation which causes the oil to go off very rapidly.

A few simple pointers will help you to prolong the life and therapeutic value of your oils, so you can get the best out of them down to the last drop.

● Always store bottles of oil in a cool, dark place, away from heat and light, with caps firmly on. Kept this way, oils should have a shelf life of 18 months. If you live in a hot climate they can be stored in the fridge – taking care to keep them well labelled and where children can't reach them. Some oils, such as benzoin, will

thicken and solidify when stored in a fridge, but will soon thin out when removed from the fridge.
● Some oils – especially the citrus oils – have very poor keeping qualities. Once opened they may only keep for three or four months. You may notice that they have a slightly fishy smell, in which case do not use. Others such as myrrh and patchouli improve with age.
● Don't allow water to get inside a bottle, as it will spoil the oil.
● Carrier oils, such as almond, grapeseed, etc., should be bought fresh regularly and used within three to six months, depending on the oil. They can be kept in the fridge to help maintain freshness, but don't use them for massage while still cold!
● Once an essential oil is added to a carrier oil its shelf life is reduced dramatically – down to just a few months. So make up small quantities of your own oils and aim to use them within three months or so. Wheatgerm oil can be added to a blend to help it keep for longer (it is a natural anti-oxidant). Jojoba oil also has very good keeping qualities, as well as being highly moisturising.

Handling essential oils

Always take great care when handling essential oils:
● Keep all essential oils out of sight and reach of children.
● Do not take essential oils internally.
● Mop up accidental spills as essential oils will leave a mark, especially on polished surfaces.
● When making up oil blends at home, ensure all bottles and utensils are very clean and dry. If preparing large quantities of oils (unlikely during pregnancy, but maybe later if you are making oil blends as presents), make sure the room is well ventilated. Essential oils can be overpowering. Always wear rubber gloves to protect the hands.
● Keep away from the eyes. If you do accidentally get essential oil in the eyes, wash them out with plenty of water. Consult a doctor is redness or irritation persists.
● Do not use essential oils neat on the skin, apart from lavender and tea-tree and then only in very tiny quantities.
● Always consult a qualified aromatherapist before using essential oils if you suffer from allergies or have any medical condition that may be affected by the use of essential oils, such as eczema, high blood pressure or epilepsy.

● If you are pregnant, use only those oils which are recommended for use during pregnancy (see pages 29–32) and never
exceed the amount stated in a recipe.

● Always think in drops when using essential oils and never be
tempted to use more drops than instructed.

● Don't self-diagnose. Always consult your GP with any medical
problem. More and more doctors are becoming sympathetic
towards complementary medicine and are perfectly happy to let
their patients try other therapies. Aromatherapy is a proven way
to help your body heal itself, but first you must know what you
are trying to heal.

6

Pregnancy massage

Pregnancy is one time in a woman's life when she needn't feel guilty about indulging herself in the occasional treat and there's no greater treat than a body massage to uplift the spirits.

Regular aromatherapy body massages throughout pregnancy – coupled with regular visits to the antenatal clinic – are a sure way of helping a mother-to-be to look and feel her best. An aromatherapy massage can help to relax the whole body and relieve the feelings of fatigue so common in the early and later parts of pregnancy. A massage is sheer bliss for aching sides, back and legs. The whole body will be toned, posture improved and any stiffness that comes with the heaviness of pregnancy can be alleviated. It can help the circulation, lower high blood pressure and improve the complexion, as well as keep the skin all over the body nourished, supple and elastic and therefore help to prevent stretch marks. Most importantly, it can help the mother-to-be to feel good about herself and keep her confidence in her looks, which is so important, as often towards the last month of pregnancy she can feel unattractive, frumpy and sexually dead (even if she doesn't seem anything like that to other people). A mother-to-be who is massaged regularly will feel good about her changing shape.

A professional massage

During pregnancy and postnatally, clients consult me for a variety of reasons. Some just because an aromatherapy massage makes them feel so good and others to treat a minor problem. Most pregnant clients book in for their first massage after they have had their first antenatal appointment, usually at around 12 weeks. I would only recommend an aromatherapy treatment after that time.

I believe in working in total co-operation with the client's doctor and midwife. This way, she can feel secure in the knowledge that everyone is working as a team for her benefit and the whole experience of pregnancy is very special.

Each client is treated totally differently. Two people visiting me might have exactly the same complaint, but might require a different approach to treatment and entirely different oils. To help me do this, before I begin a treatment I like to give a 30-minute consultation to build up a picture of the client. Some of the things I ask about are diet and exercise, relevant medical history, their general health, a history of any previous pregnancies and any allergies they may have (in case they may be allergic to any of the oils). I also need to know if there are any medical reasons why it may not be advisable to have a massage (such as a threatened miscarriage or any present illness) and any special points to take note of, such as back problems or varicose veins.

I can then advise them on the correct form of treatment, perhaps a course of aromatherapy treatments with oils to use at home as well. I always make up the oils to suit the individual and normally ask clients to keep them on for six to eight hours after a massage for maximum absorption.

It is quite normal after a first aromatherapy treatment to have a reaction. This can take the form of feeling slightly tired, or as if coming down with the 'flu, or a slight headache. These are signs that the body is throwing out toxins. It is best, on the day of an aromatherapy massage, to just relax and take it easy afterwards, to allow the full benefit of the aromatherapy treatment to work. The next day you should feel relaxed and rested. Having said this, I have never treated a mother-to-be who has experienced any side-effects whatsoever after a treatment. The people who do sometimes suffer side-effects are those that I treat for conditions such as cellulite, arthritis or stress, or conditions where there are toxins to eliminate and where strong oils are used. It is also better for clients to avoid having a large meal just before or after an aromatherapy treatment and to drink plenty of water to help flush out toxins.

When I see mothers-to-be in my aromatherapy clinics, I usually start with a back massage, getting my client to sit on the massage bed wrapped in towels, with feet resting on a stool. A towel-covered pillow is placed underneath the bump for total support. The back takes so much strain in pregnancy that quite often my clients almost purr with relief when it is massaged.

I then get the mother-to-be to lie down, supported by as many pillows as necessary to make her comfortable. Some need to be almost sitting up as they find they can't breathe properly lying down and most need pillows to support behind the knees and also the small of the back, as many women develop a hollow here in pregnancy. I then massage the legs, feet and ankles. This encourages unwanted fluid to drain. It is very common in pregnancy to have fluid retention in the lower body. I then oil and stroke the abdomen with very, very gentle movements without applying any pressure. This helps to keep the skin supple and elastic and relieve tension at the sides of the body and the diaphragm. At all times, I respect that I am actually massaging two people and it's lovely to feel the baby move as I stroke the oils over him. I am sure some babies kick out and nudge their mothers when I stop because they want me to continue.

After massaging the abdomen, the mother-to-be can change position if she wants to and I finish off with a face, neck, shoulder and head massage – unless the client dislikes oil on her hair or maybe is going out after the treatment. The oil for the face massage is individually tailored to suit the condition of the skin.

By the time the massage is over the mother-to-be is totally relaxed or sometimes asleep. I let them rest for a while before they leave my treatment rooms feeling refreshed and content or – as one mother put it – 'completely at peace with the world'.

All the mothers-to-be that I treat report that they sleep like proverbial logs after treatment and find relaxing at antenatal classes much easier.

Massaging at home

Naturally, the best person to give an aromatherapy massage is a qualified practitioner (see the Appendix for how to contact a reputable aromatherapist in your area). But it is possible to have one at home with a willing partner. Many fathers-to-be feel a very special pre-birth bond with the baby through gently massaging their partner's abdomen and feeling the baby move under their hands. Massage is also a valuable way of bringing a couple closer together, especially during the later stages of pregnancy. At this time, a woman often feels at her most unattractive, even if she isn't, and feels her husband is not interested in her as a woman. He, in turn, can feel threatened and that she is totally absorbed in the baby and may worry that making love can harm the child. Through a massage a couple can touch and remain close.

Try to get your partner to massage you regularly during pregnancy, especially if he is going to be with you during the labour. Have a well-practised set of movements planned – it's no use if he finds out you hate your feet rubbed when you get into the labour ward. He should know well in advance what you like and what is soothing, then he won't need to be instructed when it's really important. Remind him that tempers do get frayed in labour, especially at the end of the first stage, and you may not feel like talking to him.

Many men are not used to giving a massage, so it may be worth giving him, say, a foot or back massage so he can feel the variations in pressure and this will help when he massages you. It is especially useful for your partner to have a massage if he is going to be present at the birth with you (and if it isn't your partner then the person who will be) if only so that he can experience how a massage should be given and how important it is to know which movements are preferred.

Tips for home massage

If you are going to massage a mother-to-be here are a few tips:

● Collect everything you will need – such as massage oil, extra towels, etc. – before you start.
● Make the atmosphere as calm and relaxed as possible. Ensure the room is warm, dim the lights if necessary and perhaps play some soothing music. I don't advise scenting the room with essential oils, purely because, if you are using them in a massage oil, their aroma will naturally perfume the air.
● Don't do it in a hurry. If you haven't much time, just massage part of the body – say the back. If the mother-to-be is particularly exhausted the best massage is a leg and foot one. You may well find she drops off to sleep halfway through.
● After three months of pregnancy don't allow the mother-to-be to lie on her stomach.
● The ideal position for a back massage is to get the mother-to-be to sit astride a chair supported by cushions. The rest of the massage can be done on a bed covered with towels and with plenty of cushions behind the back so that she is almost sitting. As pregnancy advances, get her to lie supported by as many cushions as are comfortable for her. She may find it easier with pillows or cushions under her knees.
● When giving a whole body massage, cover her with towels and only expose the part of the body that is actually being massaged. The body temperature lowers when lying still, so she can get cold.
● Keep all movements gentle. Don't worry about being a practised masseuse. Just use any gentle movement that is relaxing and feels right. Encourage her to let you know what feels good.

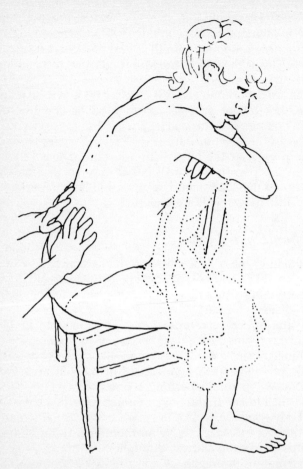

● Massage those areas where there is tension and always massage towards the heart.

● Don't press on varicose veins, just glide gently around them.

● Don't massage the mother-to-be immediately after she has had a hot bath. Although a massage feels wonderful on warm, relaxed muscles, skin that is still perspiring can't absorb oils so well. It is better to allow her to cool down a little before you begin.

● Avoid the lower abdomen and back during the first three months of pregnancy. During the rest of pregnancy, avoid deep pressure on the abdomen and lower back.

● Don't massage if the mother-to-be feels unwell or has any bleeding (in which case consult your midwife or doctor). Never massage anyone with a fever.

• Essentially it doesn't matter in which order you massage different parts of the body (see page 43 for the way in which I give a professional massage), but if you are giving a full body massage it might be easier to do the back first with the mother-to-be sitting astride a chair.

• As a rough guide, allow about 10 minutes to give a foot and leg massage, 10 minutes for a back massage and five or under for the abdomen.

Preparing a massage oil

The following recipe makes an ideal oil for massage during pregnancy:

Standard pregnancy massage oil

• Make a base oil by mixing 80 ml (4 tablespoons) sweet almond oil with 20 ml (1 tablespoon) avocado oil.

• Add 10 drops of tangerine and 5 drops of neroli oil or 10 drops of tangerine and 5 drops of lavender oil.

Back and shoulder massage

• Either the mother-to-be can lie on her side near enough to the edge of the bed for you to massage her comfortably or (for better access and results) she can sit astride a chair supported by cushions.

• With gentle upward strokes using the ready-prepared Standard Pregnancy Massage Oil (see above), glide the hands straight up either side of the spine, up over the shoulder blades, smoothing them down the side of the body and moulding them to the shape. At the waist area massage gently in circular movements to relieve the tension from overstretched ligaments.

• Always be very, very gentle in later pregnancy when massaging the lower back.

Body massage

• With the mother-to-be comfortably settled and supported on towels and pillows, stroke the oil in delicate clockwise movements around the abdomen. Remember you are massaging two people (you may well be reminded of this if the baby gives a quick kick).

• Then glide your hands to either side of the waist – or what was once the waist – and gently up and down the sides of the body. This relieves the stretching and pulling so often felt during pregnancy.

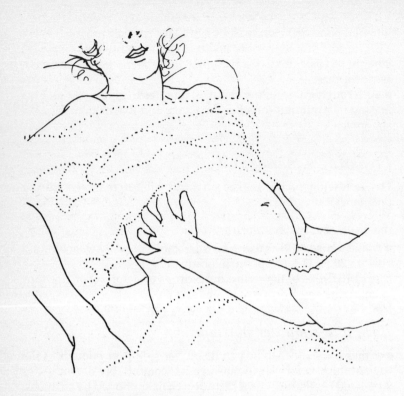

Foot and leg massage

This is a particularly good remedy for insomnia and helps to relieve fluid retention.

● The mother-to-be can sit whichever way she feel comfortable, or can lie down propped up on pillows with towels under the feet.
● Use either the Standard Pregnancy Massage Oil (see page 47) or, if the mother-to-be is having problems with aching feet and legs, you may want to use the Soothing Leg and Foot Oil (see page 55).
● Make gentle upward strokes gliding the hands from ankles to thighs, and back to the ankles again, but don't put any pressure on the downward slide. Then sweep under the foot and gently up the legs again. Try to get into a rhythm.
● Rotate the ankles first one way and then another. It also helps to flex the foot a few times as this brings a lot of relief to heavy legs.

• Massage the oil all over the feet and around the ankles. With hands cupped around one foot and fingers steadying the front of the foot, use the thumbs to make circular pressures on the sole. Gently squeeze and press the foot as though you were trying to make it into a pliable piece of dough.

After you have been massaged

Relax and enjoy the feeling of being pampered. It is best to leave the oils on to allow them to soak into the body and work properly. It can take anything from 20 minutes to seven hours for oils to work their way fully into the body via the skin, but they will be thoroughly absorbed by then, so the skin won't be left feeling at all greasy. Best of all is to have a massage just before bed, leave the oils to soak in overnight and then bathe in the morning. Then the skin will feel soft, glowing and wonderful.

Massaging your baby

Don't forget when you are applying anti-stretch mark oils on the stomach to gently feel the form of your baby. I encourage all my clients and their partners to talk to their unborn babies and the best time to do this is during the daily 'oiling session', when they can gently stroke him. If the baby is very active at night, try giving him a pre-birth massage then.

It is generally thought that in the first few weeks after birth a baby will respond to touch when he is upset, because he is used to his mother's touch. I have had several clients, who did not use aromatherapy massage with previous pregnancies, report that this time around they were convinced that after the birth their 'aroma' babies responded far more quickly to being comforted when the need arose.

7

Aromahelp
for discomforts
in pregnancy

Don't think that you will get all – or even any – of the discomforts
listed below. Every pregnancy varies from woman to woman and
even from baby to baby, but being prepared for discomforts is half
the battle. If you have any symptoms that you are particularly
worried about, consult your doctor at your regular antenatal clinics.

Back-, waist and groin ache

As pregnancy progresses, the extra weight around the stomach
really pulls at the ligaments around the waist and spine. In the
last three months, hormonal changes make the supporting joints
and ligaments relax and prepare for labour and then backache –
specially in the lower back – is more of a problem. The change in
posture can also bring niggling aches in the groin.

I generally advise women during pregnancy to:

● Take it easy. If you are aching all over it is usually a sign you are
overdoing things, so slow down.
● Take care with posture. The natural impulse as you get larger is
to stick the stomach out, but try to keep the back straight instead
of curved and try not to throw your lump out too much. Take care
not to overstrain when bending and lifting.

Aromahelp

● A regular weekly aromatherapy massage from a friend or
partner is very beneficial for strain and backache (see Chapter 6,

pages 44–49 for full details). Use the Standard Pregnancy Massage Oil (see page 47).
● Try a relaxing warm bath at the end of the day. Add 2–4 drops of lavender oil to the bath water.

Compulsory bed rest

For some women a threatened miscarriage, high blood pressure or multiple pregnancy means they have to spend much more time inactive than they'd really like to. If you are unlucky enough to have to spend some or all of your pregnancy resting in bed or on a settee, the most important thing is to calm down and take it easy.

Aromahelp

● A massage with essential oils will help you to relax. A full body massage may not be possible but get a partner or friend to give you hand, foot or facial massages (see pages 21–23).
● Don't forget to oil your stomach, breasts and thighs to help keep the skin supple.
● For a relaxing atmosphere in your room, add 2 drops of any of the following essential oils to hot water in a burner or lightbulb ring: geranium, lavender, lemon, bergamot or ylang-ylang. The vapours will fill the room.

Cramps

Cramps are very painful, shooting muscle spasms. They are very common in pregnancy – especially, it seems, in the middle of the night – but no-one really knows why. Calcium is supposed to help, so eat plenty of calcium-rich foods.

During a cramp attack, don't stretch the leg out with toes pointed. Instead rub the calf and pull the foot up towards you, then hang on to the foot until the pain passes (as your pregnancy progresses, you will have to do this sitting down with legs bent).

Aromahelp

● Massage will help. Try this massage oil:

Cramp massage oil

To 30 ml (1½ tablespoons) of almond oil, add 2 drops of lavender and 2 drops of geranium oil. Mix well.

If you have cramp most evenings or nights, then use 5 ml (¼ tablespoon) of the oil every night for a week and repeat as you need to.

Cystitis

Cystitis is the painful inflammation of the bladder and lower urinary passages which can occur more frequently during pregnancy as the growing uterus presses on the bladder. It can also mean that you have a bacterial infection. Mild symptoms can be the need to go to the toilet seemingly every few minutes but producing only a trickle and leading an uncomfortable feeling in the bladder, whilst in more severe cases it can cause burning, painful urination with fever, abdominal pain and back pain. Some women describe it as 'like trying to urinate through cut glass' and others compare it to a niggly itch that they can't reach. Either way, it is extremely uncomfortable. You may also find it is worse when you are lying down, so it's best, if you have signs of cystitis, to walk around, to sit or and keep moderately active. If you have a fever or severe pain with cystitis, see a doctor immediately. It could be an indication of kidney infection.

You can help yourself to relief by following the advice given below:

● Flush out the bladder by drinking plenty of water or lemon barley water. Current research also suggests that cranberry juice is helpful. The more you drink, the more comfortable the bladder becomes and the easier it is to urinate. Never go for too long without emptying the bladder.
● Always try to keep warm, particularly from the waist downwards. If you have an attack at night, a hot water bottle placed between the top of the legs can be comforting.
● Make sure the genital areas is washed every day with mild soap and water and rinsed well. Cystitis can be brought on by infection, so when on the toilet, wipe your bottom from front to back – rather than the other way round – to prevent infection from the bowel finding its way into the bladder.

- To avoid 'honeymoon' cystitis, brought on by intercourse and local irritation of the urethra, make sure that after making love you empty the bladder and wash the genital area.
- If you are a frequent cystitis sufferer, avoid the food or drink that you know can bring on an attack – usually alcohol or spicy foods. One client of mine get cystitis every time she drinks more than one glass of red wine.

If symptoms persist, see your doctor.

Aromahelp

- Take a warm sitz bath, to which you have added either 2 drops of lavender oil, or 2 drops of sandalwood oil, or 2 drops of bergamot oil, or 2 drops of camomile oil. Mix the oil well into the water. Soak for 5–10 minutes.
- Or have a full bath. To the warm water (never too hot), add either 2 drops of lavender oil, or 2 drops of sandalwood oil, or 1 drop of bergamot oil and 1 drop of sandalwood oil. Swish the water around to disperse the oil. Then relax and soak for 10–15 minutes in the warm water.

Take a bath with the oils mentioned above whenever you have an attack of cystitis. You may get the desire to urinate in the bath, as the warm water will ease the burning and discomfort. Don't worry if you do. I've heard doctors advise their patients to do this many times, so think of it as 'doctor's orders'.

Fatigue

Fatigue is a natural part of pregnancy. You must expect to feel tired, particularly towards the end when the extra weight and demands the baby is making on your body all conspire to slow you down.

Listen to your body. If you feel sleepy, take a nap during the day and don't feel guilty. Put your feet up whenever you can and accept all offers from friends or relations to help with the shopping, cleaning or any other chores. Make the most of it while you can.

Aromahelp

- When you need to unwind during the day or night slip into a comfortable bath with essential oils. Depending on which aroma you prefer add either:

2 drops or lavender oil, 1 drop of mandarin oil and 1 drop of ylang-ylang oil,
or
1 drop of lavender oil, 1 drop of mandarin oil and 2 drops of ylang-ylang oil.

Soak in the bath for 10–15 minutes.

Feeling faint

This quite often happens in pregnancy as the blood pressure is lower. If you feel faint, sit down and put your feet up.

Aromahelp

● Try this simple inhalation. Place 1 drop of geranium oil on a tissue or clean handkerchief. Sit back, relax and sniff as required.

Fluid retention

Fluid retention is very common in later pregnancy. Usually the first sign is the rings on your fingers becoming tight. Your ankles and feet may swell, making shoes cramped at the end of the day and you may feel very tired. Heat can aggravate fluid retention making it more of a problem during a summer pregnancy.
You should:

● Rest with your feet up – preferably higher than your head – as often as possible to allow the fluid to drain away from the ankles and feet. Avoid standing still or being on your feet for long periods of time, and take breaks if on long car journeys to move around.
● Watch your diet. Salt and sugar can both aggravate fluid retention, so check the contents of ready-made meals as they often have a high salt content. Cut down on tea and coffee.

If fluid retention is still a problem after a few simple measures, then see your doctor for a blood pressure and urine check. Don't take any diuretic pills unless prescribed by your doctor.

Aromahelp

● A foot and leg massage can really help, by pushing the fluid up and removing it as well as relieving the discomfort.

Soothing leg and foot oil

To 30 ml (1½ tablespoons) of almond oil or 30 ml (1½ tablespoons) of unperfumed oil (ask your pharmacist if unsure), add 2 drops of lavender oil and 2 drops of geranium oil.

Massage the legs and feet with this oil – you can either do this yourself or get someone to do it for you.

Starting at the ankle, massage with firm upward strokes over the knee to the upper thigh (or just massage lower leg to knee). Glide hands down and repeat.

Rotate the ankles first one way and then another. It also helps to flex the foot a few times as this brings a lot of relief to heavy legs.

Massage the feet by pressing and rubbing them. Make circular pressures with thumbs over the soles. Stroke the front of the feet firmly down from the base of the toes to the ankles and circle around the ankles.

● Footbaths can also help. For a soothing footbath add 1 drop of geranium oil and 1 drop of lemon oil to a bowl of coolish water. Soak your feet in this for as long as you need to.

Haemorrhoids or piles

Haemorrhoids are congested veins around the rectum and anal canal, which can be itchy, sore and make opening the bowels very painful. They can even bleed. They are aggravated by the pelvic congestion that results from pregnancy.

It helps to avoid getting constipated, so eat a high-fibre diet and lots of fruit and vegetables and drink plenty of water. If you are constipated, don't strain when on the lavatory as this will make the haemorrhoids worse. Medical opinion these days for anyone (not just pregnant women) is that sitting on the toilet for too long, reading magazines and waiting for something to happen, actually encourages piles. You may find it more comfortable to wipe the bottom with damp cotton wool after opening the bowels.

Aromahelp

● Take a warm (not hot) sitz bath to which you have added 2 drops of geranium oil and 2 drops of cypress oil. Soak in it for 10 minutes.

● Or soak a J-cloth or pad of cotton wool in the same solution and hold it against the back passage. You may find this easier to do while sitting on the toilet.

● Try a compress. This sounds like torture but I promise it brings wonderful relief. To a small bowl of water, add 2 drops of geranium oil and 2 drops of cypress oil. Soak a J-cloth in this mixture, then wrap the cloth around a small bag of ice cubes or small packet of frozen peas. Hold it against the anus for 1 minute (or slightly longer if you really need to). Repeat every 4 hours and after opening the bowels.

● Apply a small amount – about a teaspoon – of the following gel to the piles, after opening the bowels and whenever they are sore and itchy.

Haemorrhoid gel

To a 50 ml pot of aloe gel or any lubricating gel such as KY jelly, add 5 drops of cypress oil and 5 drops of geranium oil. Mix well.

Indigestion and Heartburn

Indigestion can occur throughout the pregnancy. Heartburn is a burning sensation in the lower part of the chest that sometimes comes with bringing up small amounts of acidy fluid. It is more common towards the end of the pregnancy.

The following tips should help:

● Look at your diet and avoid the foods that cause indigestion or heartburn – usually spicy, fried or dairy foods. Don't overeat.

● Towards the end of the pregnancy, as the baby gets larger, the stomach may be rather squashed, so it may be better to eat smaller meals more frequently.

● If it is a bad problem, you may think about food combining (i.e. not mixing foods that fight, such as protein and starch) to help the digestion. There are several books available on this subject.

Aromahelp

Use the Standard Pregnancy Massage Oil (see page 47) to gently massage to solar plexus, between the breasts and bump. Or use the following oil:

Indigestion massage oil

To 10 ml (¹/₂ tablespoon) of any carrier oil (see pages 33–35), add 2 drops of sandalwood oil, or 2 drops of orange oil or 2 drops of mandarin oil. Mix well.

Sandalwood would be the best choice if you have it. It makes an excellent massage oil to use any time you have indigestion.

Insomnia

Towards the end of pregnancy and especially in the last month, many women find it increasingly difficult to sleep, especially if the baby is active and kicking at night.

Try resting your bump on a pillow to make lying on your side more comfortable. It can also help if you increase the amount of pillows you sleep on from two to four to help breathing. Also, wear loose night clothes and cut out tea and coffee in the evening – a warm milky drink can help last thing at night.

Aromahelp

● A gentle massage before going to bed is one way to relax and sleep well. If there is no time for a full body massage, just ask a friend or partner to massage the feet (see page 48), as this is very soporific. Use the Standard Pregnancy Massage Oil (see page 47).
● A relaxing bath can help just before bed. To a warm bath, add 3 drops of lavender, mandarin or ylang-ylang oil. Swish the water to disperse the oil. Relax and soak for 10 minutes.
● Scent the bedroom to induce sleep. To a burner, diffuser or bowl of hot water, add 2–3 drops of lavender or ylang-ylang oil or a mixture of these two oils.

Morning Sickness

This is often one of the first symptoms of pregnancy. The awful feeling of nausea that comes with morning sickness, contrary to the name, can happen at any time of the day – though it is more common first thing in the morning. It can also continue well past the first three months of pregnancy.

During pregnancy the sense of smell becomes more acute. Some women find they can't tolerate even normal household smells or smells they usually enjoy, such as their favourite perfume. For this reason, it's very hard to recommend an essential oil for morning sickness and I feel there is only a limited amount that aromatherapy can do to help, but here are some general tips:

● The most important thing is to avoid all food or smells that make you feel queasy. The usual culprits are coffee, dairy foods, cigarette smoke and fried food. If cooking makes you sick, then get someone else to cook for a while.
● Avoid getting out of bed too quickly in the morning. Sit up slowly and keep still for about 10 minutes. Try to take things much more slowly during the day as well, as rushing about can bring on nausea.
● Upon waking, sip Indian or China tea very slowly. (If no-one is on hand to wait on you then take a thermos flask to bed with you with some powdered milk). Alternatively, try sipping hot water with the juice of half a lemon, or infuse a small piece of fresh root ginger in a cup of boiling-hot water (remove the ginger after five minutes and drink slowly) or add a pinch of dried ginger to a cup of hot water (do *not* use essential oil of ginger).
● When you wake, nibbling on some dry toast, plain dry biscuit or thin slices of crispy apple can help to settle the stomach.
● Don't take over-the-counter medications unless you GP has approved them and if your vomiting is severe then see your doctor.

Aromahelp

As I've already said, it is difficult to prescribe an essential oil for morning sickness, because of the aversion to a large number of scents that often comes with pregnancy. However, some women find that 1–2 drops of lemon oil in a burner or diffuser in the bedroom will help to relieve nausea. Use whenever feeling nauseous. If the feeling of sickness persists throughout the day, then try the same remedy in whatever room you happen to be in.

Nosebleeds and mucus

Nosebleeds and extra mucus, or stuffiness in the nose, are common side effects of pregnancy, due to increased blood supply to the nasal passages. They both usually end as soon as pregnancy is over, but if they continue to be a problem you should inform your doctor at your next antenatal clinic.

Aromahelp

● An inhalation will remove the pressure on the nasal passages if you have a stuffy nose, but never use this treatment if you have a nosebleed as it will make it worse.

To a bowl of hot water, add 2 drops of eucalyptus or tea-tree oil and inhale the steam for a couple of minutes.

● A facial massage can also help deal with excess mucus.

To 10 ml (½ tablespoon) of jojoba or grapeseed oil, add 1 drop of lavender oil to make a massage oil. Using this massage oil on the fingertips, press and release the fingers gently along the cheekbones. This will loosen any mucus.

● If you have a nosebleed, pinch the bottom of the nostrils quite hard for a short while – a minute or two – and it should stop. Or use the compress below. Obviously, if you have frequent or severe nosebleeds, consult your doctor.

Compress for nosebleeds

Place about 300 ml (½ pint) of very, very cold water in a bowl (add ice if necessary). Add 1 drop of cypress oil or 1 drop of lemon oil.

Agitate the water, squeeze out a J-cloth or any other clean cloth in it, then use the cloth as a compress, by laying it on the top of the nose for a few minutes. The nosebleed should stop.

Palpitations

When you have palpitations, it is medically termed as 'being aware of the heartbeat'. Palpitations can be felt as 'fluttering feelings in the chest' or sometimes as 'missing a beat'. They can be caused by drinking too much coffee or sometimes by stress. Those who are nervous are particularly prone to them. They are often wrongly described as 'a rapid heartbeat' (tachycardia). However, as a rapid heartbeat can also be caused by stress and fear, the same essential oils can help both conditions.

If you suffer from palpitations, cut down on all stimulants such as tea, coffee and fizzy drinks such as colas, but see your doctor if they are severe.

Aromahelp

- To 10 ml ½ tablespoon) of a carrier oil (see pages 33–36) add 1 drop of neroli oil or 1 drop of ylang-ylang oil. Massage this into the feet, the back of the hands or the abdomen.
- Ylang-ylang oil can also be used in a diffuser, burner or bowl of hot water to scent the room. This is very calming.

Preparing the perineal area

The perineum is the skin between the vagina and the anus. It will be stretched quite a bit during labour, so needs to be given a little help beforehand.

You should never apply essential oils to the perineum as it is a very sensitive area. During the last eight weeks of your pregnancy, gently rub it daily with ¼ teaspoon of jojoba oil. Jojoba is highly lubricating and will help the skin to become more supple and may prevent tearing during labour.

Skin problems

The skin in pregnancy varies so much from woman to woman. Some find their skin, hair and nails have never looked better and they truly 'bloom'; others suffer from greasy skin and lank hair.

If pregnancy is taking its toll on your skin, take the normal precautions, such as making sure you have a good diet (with plenty of vitamin C) and try to get as much sleep as you can.

It can really boost morale in pregnancy to get a professional pedicure or manicure to keep the nails looking good, and always keep hair well washed (either by yourself or by a friend if it gets difficult to bend over a basin in the later stages of pregnancy).

I remember I was always hot when I was pregnant and many women tell me they are the same, so the skin can often get quite clammy. Orange flower water, used in an atomiser (or a plastic version of the same thing which is quite easy to obtain at the chemist) to spray on the face, can be a real help. It can also be useful to take into hospital for when you are in labour.

Aromahelp

● Your aromatherapist can advise you on skin and hair care, depending upon your individual needs, but the massage oil below can help:

Facial massage oil
To 10 ml (½ tablespoon) of jojoba oil, add 1–2 drops of lavender, neroli or sandalwood oil.

Massage this oil lightly into the face about three times a week after cleansing. You will probably find the oil sinks in completely, but if there is any excess, blot off with a tissue. Never go to bed with an oily face as it could cause puffiness under the eyes in the morning.

See Chapter 12 for more recipes for skin care.

Sore breasts

One of the first signs of pregnancy is sore or swollen breasts that feel rather as they do before a period.

It is important to wear a well-fitting bra throughout pregnancy to give your breasts proper support. You may have to change sizes several times as they gradually swell and get larger. Get them measured professionally if you are in any doubt as to the size. You can do this in any lingerie department of a large store.

If your breasts feel very heavy and uncomfortable, wear a bra – preferably a cotton one – at nights as well.

Aromahelp

● Use the Anti-Stretch Mark Oil (see page 62) to massage the breasts. Regular use will help to avoid getting stretch marks.
● Bathe regularly in warm water to which you have added 2 drops of lavender oil or 2 drops of geranium oil. Lie back and let the water cover your breasts or soak a flannel in the water and hold it to your breasts.
● Try this compress. To 300 ml (½ pint) of water (it can be either hot or cold – whichever gives most relief), add 2 drops of lavender and 2 drops of geranium oil. Soak a cloth in the water and then hold the cloth to your breasts.

Sore or bleeding gums

Soft and bleeding gums are more common during pregnancy, again due to hormonal changes. They can also be a sign of gum disease, so do visit the dentist for a check-up and also, if you can, a hygienist to get your teeth and gums thoroughly cleaned.

Keep your teeth scrupulously clean and floss well between them each time you brush them. Making sure that you have a good intake of Vitamin C will also help.

Aromahelp

● Unfortunately, the essential oils I would normal recommend to treat sore or bleeding gums – such as clove and myrrh – are not suitable to use in pregnancy, but it may help to squeeze some lemon juice in a small glass of water and use this as a mouthwash.

Stretch marks

Stretch marks are the thin red streaks that can form on the abdomen, thighs, breasts, hips, buttocks and tops of arms during pregnancy. In severe cases they may even bleed. They are due to a weakening or breakdown of the underlying fibres in the skin. Once these fibres have been overstretched, they will not go back to normal after the weight decreases, but the marks will fade considerably from red to silver feathery lines. Those with delicate fair skin are the most vulnerable. Try to avoid putting on weight too rapidly in pregnancy. A slow gain will allow the skin time to adjust.

Aromahelp

● With aromatherapy the attitude is that prevention is better than cure. Tangerine, neroli and lavender oils have been shown to promote healthy skin cells when combined with either a moisturising cream or a massage oil. Use the recipe below, or you can use the Standard Pregnancy Massage Oil (see page 47) to help to keep the skin supple and elastic and prevent stretch marks.

Anti-stretch mark oil

To 80 ml (4 tablespoons) of almond oil and 20 ml (1 tablespoon) of avocado oil, add:

7 drops of lavender and 5 drops of neroli oil,
or
7 drops of lavender and 5 drops of mandarin or tangerine oil,
or
7 drops of mandarin or tangerine and 5 drops of neroli oil.

Apply a small amount of the oil daily and massage in gently to the hips, stomach, thighs and breasts, paying attention to any area that feels particularly taut or to previous scar tissue. This can also help to relieve the tightness and itching that comes with rapid weight gain, as in a multiple pregnancy.

● After the birth, carry on using the Anti Stretch-Mark Oil until your weight and figure get back to normal, as, surprisingly, stretch marks can occur when weight is decreasing.

Thrush

We all have a multitude of bacteria living naturally in our intestines, some of them highly beneficial to our well-being. If some of these 'good' bacteria are destroyed, then the body goes into an unbalanced state and other organisms, that also normally live harmlessly in the body, can start to overgrow and cause infection.

One such organism, a yeastlike fungus called *Candida albicans*, is responsible for the infection of the mucus membranes we know as thrush. It can affect the bowel, mouth, skin and vagina. Thrush can take hold in the vagina when the vaginal tract becomes too alkaline (it needs to be slightly acidic, just like the surface of our skin). This can happen for a variety of reasons:

● It may follow or occur during a course of antibiotics because these drugs, as well as attacking unwanted bacterial infection, can also kill off the 'good' bacteria that help to maintain the acid-alkali balance in the vaginal tract.
● Hormonal changes during pregnancy and postnatally can also upset the acid-alkali balance in the vaginal tract and increase the chances of getting it, as can the menopause and taking the contraceptive pill.
● It can occur in those with poor health whose immune systems are worn down and in those suffering from gross fatigue and stress.

The first sign is an irritating, white, thick discharge rather like cottage cheese. The vaginal tract can become red, sore and may bleed a little when touched. There may also be some pain on urinating and during intercourse.

The following advice should be helpful:

● Pay attention to your diet. Cut back on the foods that encourage thrush – anything sugary, alcohol and refined foods. Cut down on tea and coffee and it may also be wise to cut down on fruit. Eat plenty of live natural yoghurt containing lactobacillus, as this will redress the balance of friendly bacteria in the intestines. Eat foods rich in B vitamins, such as fresh vegetables and wholegrain cereals.
● Wear cotton underwear and stockings instead of tights, as thrush thrives in damp and unventilated areas.
● During an attack of thrush, don't share bath towels with anyone else, change the one you do use every day and don't use a flannel as they can spread germs.
● See your doctor if the attack is very severe and you may be given some pessaries. Essential oil treatments can be used at the same time as these.
● To prevent further attacks, use a condom during intercourse with your partner – he can re-infect you. Ensure the condoms are well lubricated. If they are too dry, the irritation will make the thrush even worse. It is also wise that your partner receives treatment at the same time as you. He can use any of the recipes below.

Aromahelp

Some essential oils, particularly tea-tree and lavender, have been shown in inhibit the growth of thrush and other fungal infections. When used in a diluted solution they can really bring relief by alleviating the itching and inflammation, soothing the infected areas and helping to treat the condition.

Thrush essential oil mix

In a small 10 ml dropper bottle (available at the chemist), add 8 mls (about 1½ teaspoons) of tea-tree and 2 ml (about ⅓ teaspoon) of lavender oil. Mix well.

Add 2–4 drops of this mixture to a warm bath and soak in the water for 10 minutes. You can also add 2–3 drops of this mixture to a basin or bidet of warm water and use this to wash the vaginal area.

Never use commercial bubble baths etc. if you have thrush, as these are too alkaline and can irritate the vagina.

● Use the following cream to soothe the delicate vulval area. Apply 3–4 times a day.

Soothing thrush cream
To 30 g (1 oz) of unperfumed cream, unperfumed gel (ask your chemist if unsure) or a pot of aloe gel, add 7 drops of the Thrush Essential Oil Mix (see above).

● As well as eating natural yoghurt to help restore the 'friendly' bacteria in their intestines, many women find that inserting a yoghurt and tea-tree-oil mixture into the vagina not only soothes and stops the intense itch, but can prevent a full-blown attack from developing.

The yoghurt and tea-tree-oil mixture is inserted into the vagina on a tampon, so this method should *never* be used in pregnancy, only postnatally when you have been told by your doctor or midwife that you may resume wearing tampons again (see **Caution** below).

From a pot of plain live yoghurt, remove enough to completely coat a slightly damp tampon. Add 1 drop of tea-tree oil and mix well into the yoghurt. Roll the tampon into this mixture, making it wet and well coated. Insert the tampon into the vagina and leave in place for 2–3 hours. Repeat as necessary. Don't use any other essential oil on a tampon but tea-tree; it is a powerful anti-fungal agent and the only oil mild enough for the very delicate vaginal tract. It must only be used in low dilutions.

CAUTION: Although I have included this tampon method in a chapter on help for problems in pregnancy, it is advisable that you do *not* insert tampons into your vagina during pregnancy. It is better that you use the external method of easing thrush given above. However, if you have a severe bout of thrush that is not being controlled by nystatin pessaries and wish to use this soothing method, it is important that you seek the advice of your midwife or doctor *before using it*.

Tampons should also not be used during the weeks following childbirth, because of infection. Again, ask your midwife for advice.

Women who use tampons should also be aware of a *rare* condition known as toxic shock syndrome. This is caused by bacteria and has been found to be more common in tampon users. It can quite rapidly lead to a feverish illness; the symptoms include fever, a rash, vomiting, a sore throat, dizziness and diarrhoea.

Your doctor should be able to give you advice on toxic shock syndrome and the use of tampons, but generally a tampon should never be left in place for more than three hours and it is best not to use them at night. Also, always use the lowest absorbency tampon you can and check that the previous tampon has been removed before inserting another.

Varicose veins

Varicose veins are purplish dilated veins that often develop in the legs, calves and even the groin in later pregnancy. They are caused by increased weight hindering the return of blood to the legs and can result in aching legs and throbbing pains.

If you already had varicose veins before becoming pregnant they may be more pronounced now, as increased weight causes pressure in the pelvic area. The good news is that if they are brought on by pregnancy, they often disappear fairly swiftly afterwards.

The following tips should help:

● Standing still or sitting with your legs crossed will aggravate varicose veins. A gentle daily walk will help the circulation, as will putting your feet up when you sit. Try to rest with your feet higher than your head as often as possible and if you have really bad veins and fluid retention, if might be a good idea to raise the end of your bed up slightly on blocks.
● Exercise the calf muscles by flexing the feet up and down. Also give the legs a really good stretch by rotating the ankles first one way and then the other.

Aromahelp

● A warm bath will help to relieve throbbing pain (never use hot water as this will aggravate varicose veins). Add 4 drops of lavender oil to the bath water and swish to disperse. Relax and soak for 10–15 minutes.
● Whenever your legs are aching, gently stroke this wonderfully cooling lotion up them:

Varicose vein leg lotion

To a 100 ml (just under ¼ pint) bottle of unperfumed lotion, add 5 drops of lemon, 5 drops of geranium and 5 drops of cypress oil. Mix well and keep the bottle in the fridge.

Never massage below varicose veins, just glide around the side of them. You could also ask your partner to rub your feet with this lotion, stretching and rotating them to aid the circulation.

8

Aromahelp for labour and birth

These days, natural childbirth has taken on a new meaning. It is no longer a taboo subject, representing mothers against doctors and the establishment. I can remember, though, not so long ago, when mothers had to seek out individual hospitals or obstetricians who would not disapprove if they did not want to be filled with pethadine or wired up to rooms of machinery during childbirth because it was considered the way of modern, safe medicine.

Today a mother is given the choice on how she wants to give birth. Views on orthodox and complementary pain relief have changed and can now work hand in hand. Hospital staff respect the mother's preference and aim to make the birth a safe but happy experience for both mother and child. Today, the same staff who can at a moment's notice help to perform an emergency Caesarean by epidural, can also, at another time, be found scenting the room with jasmine or lavender and massaging the mother's back with aromatic oils.

It is worth mentioning here that however well you plan your labour, birth is often is often a very unpredictable and dramatic event and, even with the best will in the world, it may not go quite as you wished. You may, for example, have planned a natural birth and then find yourself upset if this happens to you or feel that you have 'failed' in some way. The most important thing, obviously, is that your baby is healthy and delivered safely.

Essential oils for labour

Even if you have decided that you want the full benefits of modern medicine when you give birth, essential oils can still be of enormous help. If you want a natural childbirth they can prove invaluable. Previous chapters have mentioned their pain-relieving and calming properties. During labour some of them will be especially helpful. For scenting the labour room, choose oils with the aromas you prefer – this will be important in helping to calm and soothe you.

Feedback from my clients and from midwives confirms that women who get the best results from aromatherapy during labour are those who have used the oils during pregnancy. As one midwife put it, 'The mothers who have used the oils before know what to expect from them and are calmed by their smell as soon as they reach the unit. They don't need to waste time grasping the concept of them, whereas mothers experiencing oils for the first time still get relief from pain with the massages, but don't understand immediately that the smell of these oils can be calming at a time when they may already be in some distress.' So if you are planning to use essential oils at any stage of your labour – even if it is just for a soothing bath when you are still at home and in the first stage – then it is best to be familiar with them.

Rose

This most feminine of all oils is said to have an affinity with the reproductive system. In everyday use, it is chosen for many uterine disorders as it has a regulating, toning and cleansing effect on the uterus. For this reason, rose is highly appropriate for labour. It is a tonic to the whole system and can assist the circulation, which in turn can encourage deep and calm breathing. Rose in renowned for its anti-depressant qualities. It has a lovely, uplifting aroma that helps to calm nervous feelings.

Rose can be used alone in a massage oil, but I suggest its use in an equal blend with lavender as a massage oil. Or, if you are feeling totally extravagant, as a bath oil during the first stage.

Clary sage

Some people like to use clary sage during delivery as it is a great tension reliever, but some people can feel sleepy after using it. It can also be euphoric and a little too heady and may make everyone in the delivery room a little spaced out. It can, however, relieve pain, so use on a compress rather than in a massage oil. It is not an oil I would recommend if the mother has gas and air or has to have a general anaesthetic.

Neroli

Neroli is helpful in labour to reduce fear, apprehension and anxiety. It helps you to breathe properly, allowing you to concentrate on the slow, calm breathing techniques you have practised for labour. Just one or two drops, on a tissue to inhale or in a room spray or vaporiser, can encourage regular, rhythmic breathing.

Jasmine

Jasmine is a warm and fragrant oil that has proved to be extremely helpful during childbirth. Its analgesic and anti-spasmodic actions can help to dull uterine pain and it strengthens contractions, which in turn helps to shorten labour. It has a calming yet energising and uplifting effect on the emotions and so is an ideal oil to choose if feeling anxious, or if your confidence just needs a boost to keep you going. It can also assist breathing.

I recommend its use in a massage oil either by itself or in a blend with lavender, as the two oils work very well together. On its own it can also be used on a compress laid on the lower abdomen immediately after the birth to help expel the placenta.

Lavender

This remarkably useful oil is the one you are most likely to be offered in hospital for pain relief. Like jasmine, it is very helpful in labour, for dulling and easing uterine pain or for soothing aching legs and back. It increases the strength, but not the pain of contractions. Used in a warm bath in the first stage of labour, lavender has a relaxing and calming effect, especially on the mood swings so common at this time. It will soothe any headaches brought on by nervous tension and help dispel feelings of panic – so common in a first pregnancy – that result from the fear of the unknown.

Because of its antiseptic properties, lavender can be used in a burner, diffuser or bowl of hot water to cleanse the air in the delivery room and its antiseptic qualities will bring protection from any bugs loitering in hospital baths.

Geranium

Geranium is good for the circulation, which in turn will aid breathing in labour. It is a very balancing oil, with the same effect on the emotions, and has a lovely uplifting smell which makes it a good choice to use to scent the room during labour.

Ylang-ylang

This is a very calming oil, which is why it is recommended for labour. It is particularly helpful for those with a rapid heartbeat or who are fearful and anxious, as it is so soothing and also acts as an anti-depressant. Ylang-ylang can help to lower blood pressure and, like geranium, is a good oil to use in a burner or diffuser in the labour room.

Note: Many women, whether at home or in hospital, prefer to give birth in water. I don't recommend the use of essential oils in birthing pools, as the oils float in water and there is a very small chance that they could get into the baby's eyes. The oils are better used for scenting the room.

Preparing oils for labour

Prepare all your labour massage and bath oils in advance. Ensure each bottle is labelled with your name and what it is being used for. Keep them somewhere cool, in a plastic sponge bag to avoid any leaks, and, if you need to, keep a note in your hospital suitcase as to where they are. Hospitals always seem to have their heating systems on full whatever the time of year, so any clothes, underwear and nightwear you take to the hospital are better made of cotton. To refresh you any time, pack a bottle of orange flower water with some cotton-wool balls.

Labour day – the first stage

At last the weeks of waiting and preparation are over. During the final weeks of your pregnancy, you may well feel that your body has taken enough and you are completely fed up with the pregnant state. And, although you may be longing to see and hold your baby, you will probably feel both excited and apprehensive – or even fearful. These are perfectly natural reactions, and not just confined to those having a first baby. Birth is an overwhelming, all-absorbing experience every time.

Your contractions have started, you have had a show or maybe your waters have even broken. Whatever has occurred, your labour has started and you are on your way. Whether you are having your baby at home or in hospital, you will almost certainly – unless there are medical reasons – be encouraged to keep active until the contractions are quite strong (although that doesn't mean going out shopping for the day). Keeping moderately active is a good idea as it helps to speed up the birth and relieve pain.

Aromahelp

● If you go into labour during the early evening a bath will be very soothing, and will relieve the tension caused by the excitement and apprehension. It will also enable you to get a few hours' sleep – very important as you have a lot of work to do.

Labour bath mix
To a warm bath, add 2–3 drops of lavender oil. Swish the water to disperse the oil. Relax and soak for 10 minutes.

● Get your partner to massage you (see pages 72–74 under Advanced First Stage).
● As the contractions become stronger – whether you are still at home or in hospital – again a warm bath is a great pain reliever. If your waters have broken, check with your midwife that this is all right, as opinions vary, but many hospitals allow mothers to stay in the bath as long as they feel comfortable.

The advanced first stage

At this stage of the proceedings, whether at home or in hospital, you will now be in the very welcome and reassuring care of your midwife. During this sometimes long stage of labour, the uterine muscles are working hard at pulling up and opening the cervix. Women experience labour pains differently – some may feel pain in the lower back; others across the lower abdomen or down the thighs.

It is now, as the contractions become stronger, that along with your massage partner or willing midwife, you can put into practice all the relaxing techniques you have learnt over the past few months.

Aromahelp

● You may find that spending long periods soaking in a bath is a great pain reliever at this stage – unless of course there are medical reasons why you can't have one. Use the Labour Bath Mix given on page 72.

The following compress will also help ease pain:

Compress for lower back or abdomen

To 300 ml (½ pint) of warm water, add 2–3 drops of clary sage, jasmine or lavender oil.

Agitate well, then swish a J-cloth or other suitable cloth in the water, squeeze it out and place it on either the lower back or the abdomen. Leave for as long as you feel comfortable or until the compress loses warmth. Repeat if you need to.

● Don't just do one thing, though. Try both aromatic baths and compresses, coupled with massage (see below) and frequent changes of position. Keep moving around as much as you can during this stage of labour. It also helps to perfume the delivery room (see page 76).

Labour massage

Whenever we experience pain our natural instinct is to rub it better. Nowhere could this apply more than in labour. Deep, firm, rhythmic massage can greatly reduce and relieve labour pains, especially in the first stage of labour, when you may be still at home. By the time you go into labour, hopefully your partner will be familiar with how you like to be massaged. Get him to practise the movements below well before arriving in the delivery room. Massage in labour is without doubt a great relief; with essential oils it is even better. It is courteous always to let the midwives know if you intend to use essential oils in your birth plan.

If you have no-one to accompany you to the hospital to give you an aromatherapy massage and you would like to use essential oils for your birth, find out well in advance the policy in the delivery unit. Enquire as to how many of the midwives use essential oils. If no-one who is sympathetic or familiar with them is certain to be on duty when you give birth, discover if others will understand your needs and be willing to massage you and prepare a room oil or compress if you want one. You will probably find someone who is more than happy to help you, but it is worth checking in advance.

How to give a massage during labour

If you will be massaging a mother-to-be, these are all comforting movements for labour:

• Deep, firm circular pressure around the lower back will be a help. Press the heel of your hand into the lower back of the mother-to-be.

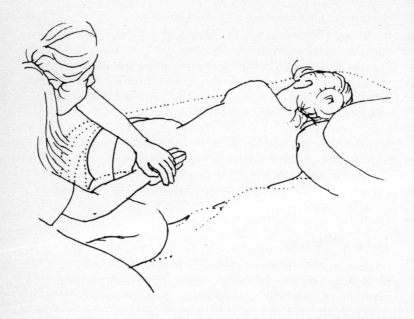

• Pressure in the centre of each buttock with the thumbs helps. Press and release several times.

• Firm pressure with the heel of your hand in her sacral area (the area below the spine) brings comfort. Massage firmly in circular movements. This is a movement that you will probably find she will want to keep coming back to throughout her labour.

• The mother-to-be may feel like sitting astride a chair (as she did in pregnancy massage) so the back and shoulders can be massaged easily, or she may want to change her position frequently. If she is comfortable on all fours, rocking gently from side to side may give relief in this position. Kneel behind her and massage in gentle circular movements down the sides of the abdomen from where the top of the bump begins to the thighs and up again. Repeat this for as long as she wants.

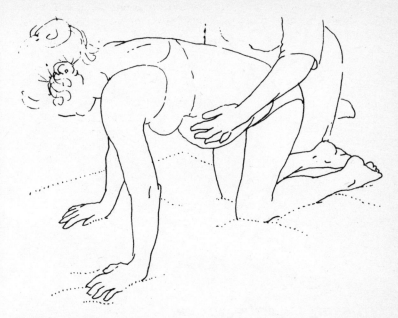

● Massaging her feet, by pressing quite firmly into the soles with circular movements, is very comforting. Use one hand to grip the top of the foot over the instep to steady it; use the other hand on the same foot, pressing firmly into the middle of the sole. Make circular movements, varying the pressure. Squeeze and release the foot. These movements should all be repeated several times.
● Still with one hand steadying the foot, press with the thumb of the other hand up and down the foot in an imaginary line. Press and release, varying the pressure and time spent on each foot according to her wishes. This feels good if the press/release action is done in circular movements.
● Still on the feet, with both hands well oiled, massage all over the top and sole of the foot and lower leg, letting the fingers circle around the ankles.

Labour day massage oil

To a 50 ml bottle of almond oil, add 6 drops of lavender and 6 drops of jasmine oil. Jasmine is quite indulgent to use as it is so expensive. If you can't afford jasmine, just use lavender on its own.

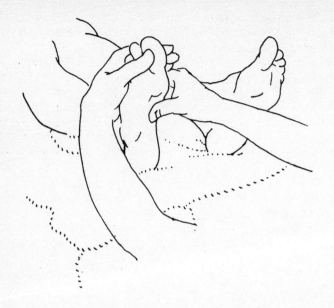

Perfuming the delivery room

Essential oils in the delivery room will help to keep the mother and everyone around her sane. For the baby, to come into the world into a sweetly scented room which is relaxed, welcoming and happy, must be the perfect way to be born.

Essential oils will also help to kill airborne bacteria and any stale smells or fuggy odours in the room and help the mother to feel calm, relaxed and happy. But take care. They are very strong and you don't want the midwife floating around the room in a trance.

Oils for the delivery room

To a bowl of hot water, add 3 drops of your favourite oil or a mix of two of the following – lavender (relaxing and antiseptic), bergamot (a great anti-depressant), geranium (as it is very uplifting) or lemon (very refreshing and good if the mother is tired after a long labour).

The transition stage

The transition stage is at the end of the first stage of labour, when the cervix has not yet fully opened and you have been told not to start pushing – although you may want to.

During the transition stage, some women find they begin to shake – especially their legs. It can be helpful if your (by now long-suffering) partner can massage your legs quite firmly, as this seems to steady them. But be warned – this is a very unpredictable and dramatic stage of labour and you may find you don't want anything to do with anyone. Don't worry if you shout and lose your temper with anything that moves – including your partner. This is all quite normal and the medical staff are quite used to it. In fact it's a sure sign that the second stage is imminent.

Aromahelp

● Some women find a cloth soaked in cool water wiped over the face and neck refreshing and calming.

Add 2 drops of rose, neroli or lavender oil to a bowl of coolish water. Soak a cloth or flannel in this and use it to mop the face.

The second stage

In the second stage of labour the cervix is fully dilated. The feel of the pains changes as the intense urge to push takes over. Calm, controlled breathing will help you over the top 'wave' of the contractions and will mean you have plenty of puff left to push with. If you find your breathing becoming erratic, sniff one or two drops of neroli on a tissue to calm you and prevent overbreathing. In between contractions, *try* to relax. It helps as you feel the next contraction coming to imagine the beginning of the pain as being like, say, a large approaching wave. Imagine your body is in total control of this wave. As the pain increases visualise the wave gradually rising to full height, reaching its peak and being held there briefly; then letting go, slowly falling to a flat level and tapering off at the water's edge, as the pain decreases and fades away.

Aromahelp

● Massage can still be soothing, but you will probably be too busy for one at this stage of labour.
● A calming cloth for your partner to dab your face with will probably be very welcome.

To a bowl of warm water, add 2–3 drops of lavender oil. Dip a J-cloth or other suitable cloth into the water and use to mop up any perspiration or just to give a soothing dab to the face.

● Place 1–2 drops of mandarin, petitgrain, neroli, ylang-ylang or geranium oil on a tissue and inhale when needed.

This may make your breathing easier and will certainly make you feel more cheerful. If you find your breathing is becoming erratic at this stage, then neroli oil is particularly recommended, as it is very calming and will prevent what is known as over-breathing, which is when gaspy breaths release carbon dioxide too quickly, making you feel dizzy and panicky with tingling face and limbs.

● Add to a bowl of hot water in the delivery room 2–3 drops of neroli, ylang-ylang or geranium oil. This will give a calming scent to the room. Ensure that the bowl is placed somewhere where it will not interfere with the proceedings.

The birth and third stage

All the past hours' work and effort seem forgotten as a somewhat slippery baby is placed on your abdomen. You will probably feel so overwhelmed that the third stage of labour – the delivery of the placenta – will probably go unnoticed by you. Relax and enjoy these moments of getting to know one another. You will always remember them.

Aromahelp

● When the baby has been delivered, a compress can help expel the placenta. This is more likely to happen at a home delivery.

To a bowl of warm water, add 2–3 drops of jasmine oil. Agitate the water well, wring out a J-cloth or other suitable cloth in it and place this compress over the lower abdomen. As the compress loses heat, replace with another. Leave in position until the placenta is delivered.

● After you have drunk the obligatory cup of tea and the two of you have been washed and tidied up you will probably be expected to sleep for a while. I was always far too excited to sleep after giving birth. If this happens to you, so you don't become too keyed up, sprinkle a few drops of neroli or lavender oil on to a tissue and inhale the aroma. Then just lie back on the pillow, close your eyes and relax. You might even be able to get some sleep.

9

Postnatal care and adjusting to motherhood

Along with the relief that the labour is all over and, hopefully, all is well, there may be some minor discomforts after the birth. After all, your body has taken a substantial battering. Aromatherapy can help you in conjunction with whatever help you receive in the hospital or from your midwife. In fact, natural products are regaining popularity in maternity units. But if in doubt over using anything, first check with your midwife. Remember to take your postnatal aromatherapy kit with you to the hospital.

Healing the perineum

If the perineum (the skin between the vagina and the anus) is sore or has stitches after an episiotomy during the birth, you are bound to feel somewhat tender and essential oils can help.

Aromahelp

● As soon as your midwife agrees, add essential oils to the bath or bidet. The mixture below will help to prevent any infection, heal wounds and encourage new skin to grow. Use the formula even if you don't have stitches as it will help to prevent infection in the days following the birth.

To a warm bath, add 2 drops of lavender and 2 drops of cypress oil. Swish the water to mix the oil in. Relax and soak for 10–15 minutes.

Use this up to three times a day while soreness persists. These oils will give great relief.

Caesarean delivery

After a Caesarean you must expect to feel tired; not only do you have a baby to look after, but you are also recovering from an operation. Allow yourself extra time to get back to normal.

Don't compare yourself to other Caesarean mothers. For every one who leaps out of bed and walks with a straight back three days after delivery, there will be 10 others who will only be able to shuffle along bent double, clutching their wound across their lower abdomens. Everyone has their own rate of recovery, so don't worry. Most mothers are able to walk with a straight back by the end of the week, but you should give yourself at least six months to get really fit again.

Please don't spend time worrying if your birth didn't go as you planned it to, or feel that you have 'failed' because you have had a Caesarean. No-one is judging you apart from yourself.

Aromahelp

• As soon as you are allowed to take a bath, add 4 drops of lavender oil to the warm (never hot) water. Swish to disperse the oil. Relax and soak for 10–15 minutes. Lavender will help you relax and help your wound heal more quickly.

Postnatal blues

It is quite normal to feel tired and weepy for a couple of days after the birth. This is often called 'third-day tears' or 'milk blues', as it happens with the arrival of breast milk. Once again, the hormones are to blame for this, so don't be alarmed if the smallest thing makes you burst into tears.

It is also a bit of a shock for first-time mothers to have to cope with leaking breasts, a sore bottom and all that that entails and – if all that weren't enough – a baby as well! It would be enough to make anyone cry. Usually these postnatal blues clear up after a few days and it's some assurance that they are never quite as bad with a second baby – if only because you know what to expect.

It is also worth bearing in mind that the days leading up to and just after the birth were probably quite an excitement – even if some of the proceedings were not that pleasant – and you will have received a tremendous amount of attention from medical staff, friends and family. Then, suddenly, you are home on your own, and looking after your baby is all up to you. A week or so after the birth of my first child I remember thinking I would never be able to do anything on the spur of the moment again. I was actually quite scared. I didn't realise that, although the responsibilities that come with being a mother would always be there, a child isn't always going to be a helpless babe-in-arms.

Talking to friends over the years, we have all come to the same conclusion, and that is that no-one prepares you or tells you what it's like to suddenly be so totally responsible for a tiny human being, who has been part of you for the last nine months but who you now have to get to know all over again. As well as the excitement and the love that brings, it can also be very frightening.

Aromahelp

● An aromatic bath will help to chase away any low feelings, so utilise any offers to help to look after the baby and take yourself off to the bathroom. Enjoy the freedom of being able to lie in the bath without looking like a hippo any more and without a pair of feet pressing on your ribs from the inside. If you have time, wash your hair as well. So many mothers say they feel better afterwards.

To the bath water (warm, never hot), add up to 5 drops of any of the following: ylang-ylang, bergamot, jasmine, neroli or clary sage oil. These are all oils that can help to lift your mood and make you feel more relaxed and cheerful.

Swish the water to disperse the oil. Relax and soak for 10–15 minutes.

● Some hospitals and midwives advise showers rather than baths for a few days after birth. If you have been advised to shower, wash as normal then add 2–3 drops of ylang-ylang, bergamot, jasmine, neroli or clary sage oil to a wet sponge and rub over your body whilst breathing in the vapours.

● If you can't bathe or shower, sprinkle 1–2 drops of either ylang-ylang, bergamot, jasmine, neroli or clary sage oil on to a tissue and sniff the uplifting aromas. Take care to keep the tissue away from the baby.

● If you really are suffering after the birth, there is a very special pick-me-up using oil from different parts of the orange tree (neroli from the flowers, petitgrain from the leaves and twigs, and orange from the fruit). It is particularly helpful for those suffering from postnatal depression as the very wholeness of the tree helps to make them feel complete.

Special pick-me-up

Either:
To a warm bath, add 2 drops of neroli, 2 drop of petitgrain and 2 drops of orange oil,
or
Make a very special massage oil, by adding 2 drops of neroli, 2 drops of petitgrain and 2 drops of orange oil to 50 ml (2½ tablespoons) sweet almond oil.

Postnatal fatigue and adjusting to motherhood

Sometimes a mother can continue to feel emotionally and physically drained for quite a while after the birth and unable to concentrate on even day-to-day tasks. With the baby taking all her time, life seems all baby and the days take on a pattern of complete non-achievement.

Before the birth we can joke about the prospect of broken nights but no-one really knows what it's like until they experience it. To be woken at two or four in the morning, especially when someone next to you is snoring their head off, is not fun. A small tip here – I really do recommend keeping a baby that is on regular night feeds in his or her cot beside your bed. The baby can then be picked up and fed without you having to get out of bed and it's also comforting for both of you to be near each other.

If this is your first baby, you may wonder how you will ever have the time or energy again to resume life as it was before, but take heart. Your body has just completed several months of the most important job it will ever do, so do give yourself a pat on the back.

Here are a few tips:

● Take time to recover at your own pace – not someone else's. If you are planning to go back to work again, make sure you feel really fit enough and are happy with the childcare arrangements. I see many women in my treatment rooms who have gone back to work too early and are feeling run-down and tired.
● Forget the housework. If the cobwebs have cobwebs it doesn't matter and if anyone else in the house is bothered about it, direct them to the cleaning materials. Gratefully accept all offers of help with the chores.

- Look after yourself, eat a well-balanced diet and allow yourself time to rest with your feet up during the day while the baby sleeps. If you have other children, keep them occupied in the same room that you are in – even if it is just watching the television – so that you can keep an eye on them and don't have to keep rushing out to see that they are up to, which is totally exhausting.
- Make sure you get exercise and fresh air, even if it is just taking the baby out for a walk with the pram every day (which is good for him too). Research has shown that exercise can release hormones that ward off melancholy feelings and depression.
- As soon as you can, get out with your partner again, even if it's just for an hour.
- Give yourself a treat – get your hair done, buy something new to wear, ask a friend to lunch (preferably one who will arrive at your house with the entire contents of a deli counter).

Aromahelp

An aromatherapy massage using oils with tonic properties will help you get back to normal. Not only will it help you to relax and feel good, but it will keep the skin on the stomach, legs and breasts well moisturised, which will encourage suppleness and tone while your weight is returning to normal. It will also encourage restful sleep – even between night feeds. One desperate and tired mother reported the best night's sleep she'd had for five years after a massage. In many Eastern countries, women routinely receive massage after childbirth to help the abdomen get back to normal.

Obviously it is better to have an aromatherapy massage from a professional, but the next best thing is one from a willing partner or friend. Follow the basic guidelines for pre-pregnancy massage (see page 21), but avoid the abdominal area altogether if there is any tenderness or if there is still postnatal bleeding. Don't massage anywhere near a Caesarean scar.

The back massage will be particularly appreciated, as the back is under a lot of stress and strain during pregnancy and the shoulders can really ache after breast- or bottle-feeding, especially with a heavy baby. Ensure you are well supported with cushions when you breast-feed.

Use the following massage oil:

Postnatal massage oil

To 25 ml (1¼ tablespoons) of carrier oil (see pages 33–35), add 3 drops of lavender, 3 drops of rosemary and 3 drops of geranium oil, or try a mix of any of the following oils: petitgrain, geranium, mandarin, rose, bergamot, ylang-ylang, lavender or rosemary.

If you are breast-feeding use only 1–2 drops of essential oil to every 5 ml (1 teaspoon) of carrier oil, as the oils are very strong and can pass through into the breast milk.

● If you are having trouble sleeping slip into a warm bath before bed. Add 3 drops of either lavender, marjoram or Roman camomile oil to the water. Alternatively, try any of the oils recommended for postnatal blues, i.e. ylang-ylang, bergamot, jasmine, neroli or clary sage.

Swish the water to disperse the oil. Relax and soak for 10–15 minutes.

● For a refreshing morning bath which will set you up for the day, add 2–3 drops of either geranium or bergamot oil and 2–3 drops of rosemary oil to the warm water. Swish the water to disperse the oil and soak as usual for 10–15 minutes.

● You can use oils around the house to scent the rooms.

To a bowl of hot water, a fragrancer or a burner, add 2–4 drops of any of the recommended postnatal oils, i.e. petitgrain, geranium, mandarin, rose, bergamot, ylang-ylang, lemon, lavender or rosemary. All of them are refreshing, but a particularly cheering and lovely blend which you may want to try is geranium and lemon.

Postnatal depression

Many women suffer from postnatal blues or fatigue, symptoms that with time and rest usually fade after a few weeks. But in true postnatal depression the feelings of fatigue, exhaustion through lack of sleep and anxiety are joined by other physical and emotional problems, which can range from fears about being a 'bad mother' to resentment towards a partner, sexual anxieties or feeling a failure if you can't breast-feed. Sometimes these problems don't appear until many months after the birth and can have their roots in a wide variety of causes.

Often they are birth-related. Some women are disappointed and unhappy at the way the delivery went and are left feeling unsatisfied, because they think their performance at the birth wasn't up to the expectations they'd set for themselves. One woman described this feeling as one of utter desolation inside. Another said she couldn't get over the disappointment of having to have a Caesarean. Someone else felt that after what she described as two physically and mentally unsatisfying births, she had to have another child to experience birth satisfaction. She did this with her third baby and then said that she felt complete.

If you have any such worries about yourself or your baby talk to your midwife or doctor. They are there to help you and they are thankfully now spotting postnatal depression earlier than in the past, before it becomes a long-term or severe problem.

It also helps to talk over your fears with other mothers, many of whom experience the same feelings to a greater or lesser degree.

Aromatherapy has a part to play in postnatal depression. If you can, see an aromatherapist as well as your doctor.

10
Breast-feeding

It must be the most natural thing in the world for a mother to put her newly born baby to her breast. Breast milk is a perfect, balanced food for a baby and it seems a terrible shame not to use it, especially as it's free. There are all kinds of other advantages in breast-feeding too, such as increasing the bond with your baby.

During the first few days after birth the breasts produce a watery fluid, colostrum, which contains antibodies that can protect the baby from infection. Even if you decide to give up breast-feeding after a few weeks, you will still have given your baby a good start by passing on these antibodies through breast milk.

Increasing the milk supply

Sometimes the breast will not provide the constant supply of milk you were hoping for and often, especially with new mothers, breast-feeding isn't as easy as you might have expected it would be. In fact, both you and your baby have to 'learn' how to do it, which can take quite a few days.

The following tips may help:

● Try to keep a relaxed attitude about feeding, as it won't benefit either you or the baby if you get tense and it can hinder the 'let-down reflex', which is the tingly feeling in and around the nipple that indicates the milk is ready to flow. This sensation has been described as feeling rather like the nose does just before you sneeze. If can feel unpleasant at first but settles down to a light tingle after the first few weeks.
● The more you put the baby to your breast the more milk you will produce – it's what's known as supply and demand. During the early days it will seem as if your breasts have taken on a new status in life!

● Don't be discouraged. Just let the baby feed whenever he or she needs to and you will soon establish a good supply. Breast-fed babies will need feeding more often than bottle-fed babies.

● Don't feel this is how breast-feeding will be all the time. It isn't. You may not believe that when you are trying to cope with heavy leaking breasts and elephant-sized bras, but after the first few weeks everything settles down, such as the size of the breast and any lumpiness. They will stop leaking and you will be able to put the baby to the breast at any time without fuss or bother.

● Don't get too tired, as this will affect the amount of milk you produce. Try and rest as much as you can and snatch sleep when the baby sleeps. If this just happens to be mid-afternoon, don't feel guilty about it.

● As a bonus, this is the one time in your life when you can eat pretty much what you want, as you will use up plenty of calories supplying the baby with milk and still lose the weight gained during pregnancy.

● You will need to take in plenty of fluid. I found that a large glass of spring water half an hour before each feed worked well, plus another glass afterwards. Drinking fennel tea is also renowned for increasing the milk flow.

● Wear a comfortable bra day and night to support the breasts, and until the milk supply settles down you may need to wear disposable breast pads as the milk does leak a little.

● If you have continuing problems, contact La Leche League or the National Childbirth Trust for the telephone number of the nearest counsellor. They can supply help and advice as well as loaning breast pumps (see Appendix for addresses).

Aromahelp

● Use the Standard Pregnancy Massage Oil (see pages 47, 62) daily on the breasts. This will help to keep the breasts supple and prevent stretch marks. Even if you didn't get these during pregnancy, the breasts may still be susceptible to them due to their increased or fluctuating size.

Continue to use twice daily until your breasts return to normal size or until after you discontinue feeding altogether.

Remember, though, to wash any oil off the nipple before feeding, or clean with moistened cotton wool and then pat dry. Medical opinion is that the nipples should not be washed too frequently when breast-feeding, but obviously it's best not to have any gel or cream on the nipple before you feed. This also applies to any creams you may have been given by the doctor.

Engorged breasts

Every woman who has breast-fed remembers the feeling of waking with rock-hard, aching breasts. The best cure is to feed the baby, but as engorgement usually occurs during the first week of breast-feeding, it may mean that a very new, sleepy baby won't be able to empty each breast completely. Also, in the beginning, the breasts can become full and lumpy very quickly, perhaps well before the baby needs another feed. Your midwife might suggest expressing the milk with a pump – this may happen if the baby is in the special care unit.

Aromahelp

● Try taking a hot bath with 2 drops of lavender and 2 drops of geranium oil added to the water. Swish to disperse the oils, then lie back and let the water cover your breasts or soak a flannel in the water and hold it to your breasts. You will find this relieves the pressure and decongests the breasts.
● Also try using a compress. A hot compress will relieve pressure and a cold compress will reduce swelling, so use whichever is most suitable.

To 300 ml (½ pint) of either hot or cold water, add 2 drops of lavender and 2 drops of geranium oil. Soak a clean cloth in the water, squeeze it, and then hold it to the breasts. You can then try to gently express some milk.

Sore nipples

Sometimes the baby may not take the whole of the nipple and surrounding area (the areola) into his mouth when feeding, but just suck at the nipple. This will not only make him frustrated at not getting enough milk, but will make you very sore and you may get cracked nipples, which doesn't make for a happy experience for either of you.

Ask your midwife to help you position the baby properly. Don't worry about this – nearly every mother needs help with breast-feeding at first. Nipple shields that the baby can suck through when he feeds (available at any chemist) will also help until the soreness has gone.

Aromahelp

● If you have any soreness, make up the following:

Sore nipple gel
To 20 ml of aloe gel, add 3 drops of rose and 1 drop of benzoin oil,
or
To 20 ml of aloe gel, add 10 ml (¹/₂ tablespoon) of a calendular carrier oil.

Apply the gel to the nipples and surrounding area after feeding the baby. Remember to wipe or wash the nipples to remove any remaining gel before feeding again as babies must not get essential oils in their mouths. This also applies to any cream, gel or lotion that you put on your breasts – even if it has been given to you by your doctor.

Mastitis

Milk blocking the ducts can lead to lumpy breasts or mastitis, when the breasts become hot and inflamed. Don't stop breast-feeding if this happens – the breasts need to be emptied – but do speak to your doctor or midwife, particularly if you are feeling unwell, because the breasts may have become infected.

11
Getting back into shape

There are a few lucky women who sail through their pregnancy and labour and effortlessly resume pre-pregnant life again with figures and complexions that are seemingly quite untouched by any of the hormonal upheaval of the past nine months. But for the other 99 per cent of us, now is the time that we need a little help boosting our post-baby morale.

Because the body works as a whole, everything we do to one part will have an effect on the entire body. So after the baby is born, diet, exercise, rest, calmness of mind and a simple beauty routine will all work together, however gradually, to help you feel totally restored and get back your confidence. But don't push yourself too hard. Let your body take its own time to get back into shape.

Aromahelp

● Throughout the three months after the birth, try to book in with an aromatherapist for regular treatments, or ask a friend or your partner to give you regular massage, even just a foot massage (see pages 21–22).
● Keep on with your essential oil baths, experimenting with the oils (but remember to use only four drops in the bath if you are breast-feeding).
● Also keep using Anti-Stretch Mark Oil (see page 62) on your body while it is returning to normal, as you can still get stretch marks after the birth when your body is decreasing in weight.

Getting your figure back into shape

Do not expect your body to spring back to its pre-pregnancy state immediately after the birth. It usually takes about 3–4 weeks for the uterus to gradually return to its normal size and this is one of the things your doctor will check at your six-week postnatal appointment. However, the stretch muscles and skin of your abdominal area will need both time and exercise to recover completely. Expect to carry excess weight around your hips, thighs and upper arms for a while. You may also suffer from fluid retention – which will soon go – and cellulite due to the hormonal change. Just remember that it took you nine months to get to the size you were for the birth of your baby, so don't expect to get back into shape again in nine days. With time and a few simple measures you will.

Diet

● Don't vow to starve yourself back into your jeans within six weeks. You will probably feel tired in the weeks after the birth and now more than ever need to regain your strength, so a low-calorie intake is the last thing your body needs, especially if you are breast-feeding, as you will need calories to produce a good supply of milk. One of the bonuses of breast-feeding, though, is that it helps the body get back into shape naturally. If you diet, you will not feel well. If you don't feel well you will not look well and you could become trapped in a vicious circle.

● Everyone recovers their energy at a different rate, but give yourself at least three months. Just be careful about what you eat in what I call the 'after-delivery recovery period'.

● Think of your diet in terms of a way of life, rather than as slimming. Whether you are breast-feeding or not, try to eat a well-balanced diet. You can lose weight without starving or depriving yourself of the odd chocolate bar. Just making a few simple changes to your eating habits will help:

● Aim for a good, balanced diet – lots vitamin-rich fruit and leafy green vegetables; plenty of low-fat protein foods, such as chicken, fish or pulses; yoghurt; carbohydrates, such as cereals, whole-grain bread and potatoes. Remember that carbohydrate foods are not fattening in themselves; it is just the sugar, jam or butter often eaten with them that pushes up the calorie content.

● Try to cut back on overall fat intake (by trimming fat off meat and avoiding oily or fried foods, etc.) and obviously sugary foods as well.

● Salt can contribute to fluid retention, so cut back on salt intake. Try herbs instead or a salt substitute for flavouring.
● Ready-prepared or processed foods will seem like a godsend just now, but do try to limit them. Check the contents list on the packets for salt, sugar and 'hidden' fats, as well as for unwanted additives.
● Drink plenty of water. Apart from the extra fluid breast-feeding mothers need, we all need at least eight glasses a day to flush out the system and keep skin clear and well hydrated.
● If you are starving hungry (and you will be quite a lot of the time if your are breast-feeding), snack on fruit or live yoghurts in between meals, rather than biscuits, sweets or cakes. If you normally consume chocolate or biscuits, aim to be realistic and limit them, rather than initially cutting them out altogether.

Exercise

● To help you recover fully from the birth, a certain amount of exercise is essential, not just to burn up calories and tone you up, but to improve your general well-being and help you feel less tired. Exercise increases the blood circulation, which in turn will help the condition of the skin.
● Choose exercise that can fit in with your daily routine – if you went to a gym or exercise class before the birth, then take it up again (once your doctor or midwife agrees you are ready and you feel strong enough) – or your exercise could be as simple as regular walking or pushing the pram. If you have no-one to look after the baby while you attend a regular exercise class, then try to find one in your area that welcomes babies too or take it in turn to babysit with another mother, so you both get the chance for an hour off every so often. Many sports centres and swimming pools offer special postnatal sessions for new mothers.
● In the early days after the birth don't neglect pelvic floor and abdominal exercises. Strong abdominal muscles help prevent low backache and pelvic floor exercises are vitally important to help stretched muscles around the vagina, bladder and anus to tone up again. Neglect them and you could develop stress incontinence – a bladder that can leak when you sneeze or run for the bus, etc. Tightening up these muscles will also mean that making love is more enjoyable – a good enough reason on its own. So however busy you are, aim to take some time every day for doing sit-ups, pelvic floor exercise or any other form of exercise that will tone up the stomach and pelvic floor. Even as little as 10 minutes a day, done regularly, will make a difference.

Body creams and lotions

In my aromatherapy treatment rooms I make up a variety of moisturising and nourishing body and hand creams for my clients. Unlike most beauty products on the market, these work on individual skin problems, right down to the lower layer of the skin. At home, too, you can benefit from individually tailored products by using unperfumed creams and adding the essential oils for your skin type.

Making up body creams

● When buying unperfumed creams or lotions, make sure they don't contain lanolin as it can aggravate skin rashes. Ask your local pharmacist to recommend one if unsure (or to find one by mail order, refer to the Appendix at the back of this book).
● If the cream is in a plastic bottle, you will need to buy some glass jars (ask your pharmacist), as essential oils don't react well with plastic. Sterilise the jars before use – using sterilising fluid – and make sure they are dry by putting them in a low oven. Also sterilise a small thin-stemmed plastic utensil for mixing the creams, or boil a coffeespoon for five minutes to sterilise it.
● When making up body creams at home, I suggest you stick to a 1 per cent dilution of the essential oils. For example:

A 1 per cent dilution of 50 g (2 oz) cream would contain 12 drops of essential oil.
A 1 per cent dilution of 30 g (1¼ oz) cream would contain 7 drops of essential oil.

● Following the above directions for quantities, squeeze the cream into the jar and add the essential oils. Stir very well to make sure the oil is distributed evenly and don't forget to label the jar afterwards.

I think the fragrance is more alluring when just a single oil is used instead of a blend of several. Any of the following oils will make delicious-smelling body creams: ylang-ylang, mandarin, geranium, rose, jasmine, neroli, lavender, petitgrain and sandalwood (see pages 94–95, under Body Scrubs, for which are suitable for particular skin types).

Use creams as often as you wish to, but preferably at least once a day.

Body scrubs

As I've already stated, the skin is one of the organs of elimination for the body and when it is clogged up, the pores have to work much harder to get rid of unwanted toxins and waste. The skin will also be more receptive to oils or creams if it is not congested with dead cells, which can linger, giving skin a sallow or dull tone. By removing dead cells the skin is thoroughly cleansed and the pores unclogged of dirt, so the skin can breathe again. Skin brushing or using exfoliating scrubs gives nature a hand in this process, leaving the skin glowing and soft.

How often you use a body scrub will depend on how you think your skin looks and the time you have available, but aim for at least once a week as it will help a sluggish circulation. If you have had a Caesarean, you must keep well clear of the abdomen until the scar and any internal bruising have healed.

There are many body scrubs available commercially, but most tend to be expensive and too abrasive. The gentle scrub below is easily made at home, with essential oils added to suit the condition of the skin. It will leave the body soft and glowing.

Basic scrub mix

Mix together 100 g (4 oz) oatmeal and 100 g (4 oz) ground almonds. If you only have whole almonds, first remove the skins – make sure they are dry or they will go off when stored – and grind in a food processor.

Store the mixture in a glass jar and keep the lid on to keep dry.

Body scrub

● Place 1–2 tablespoons of the Basic Scrub Mix (see above) in a small basin. Add 4 drops of chosen essential oil – either any recommended postnatal oil or one recommended for your skin type:

Recommended postnatal oils: benzoin, clary sage, Roman camomile, marjoram, rosemary and grapefruit.
For dry or sensitive skin: rose, sandalwood and neroli are best. Other suitable oils are Roman camomile, jasmine and ylang-ylang.
For normal skin: lavender, geranium and neroli are best. Other suitable oils are sandalwood, rose and jasmine.
For oily skin: ylang-ylang, geranium, lemon, lavender and cypress are best. Another suitable oil is sandalwood.
For allergic skin: camomile and sandalwood.

• Add ¹/₂ teaspoon of jujube or almond oil. Mix to a paste. Add more jujube or almond oil if it is too stiff.
• Bath or shower as normal, pat yourself nearly dry and then with damp skin, rub the paste all over the body starting at the feet and working upwards (it is best to do this while standing in the bath or shower). Work the mixture into the body with gentle circular movements, avoiding any areas that are sore (such as breasts or nipples), scarred or near to varicose veins. Work well into any areas of cellulite or dry skin.
• Rinse off well and the skin should be soft and glowing.

Getting rid of cellulite

The body tends to use the hips and thighs as a dumping ground for surplus wastes and toxins, giving rise to the familiar orange-peel skin known as cellulite. The skin is dimply and lumpy, usually feels cold to the touch and can be quite painful when pressed. Women tend to accumulate cellulite at times of hormonal fluctuations and therefore during pregnancy are far more prone to it.

Cellulite can affect those who are thin as much as those who are overweight. It occurs when the body's elimination processes aren't functioning properly. As well as hormonal changes (which explains its appearance at puberty, pregnancy and the menopause) other causes of cellulite are constipation, lack of exercise, fatigue and filling the body with toxins over a long period, such as too much alcohol, tobacco, tea, coffee, animal fats, dairy products, etc. Cellulite also goes hand in hand with having poor circulation and poor lymphatic drainage.

An aromatherapist can help with cellulite, but I wouldn't recommend treatment until six months after the birth. To make concentrated effort to remove cellulite involves a quite strict detoxification diet, plus possibly a lymph drainage programme, and this is not advisable until this time – especially if you are breast-feeding.

But, in the meantime, there are certain measures you can take to reduce it.

• Exercise and improving your diet are the first steps. Follow the instructions given above in the sections on diet and exercise (see pages 91–92). All the measures mentioned there will help – such as cutting back on fat intake and drinking plenty of water to flush toxins out of the system. It is also important to get some form of regular exercise. It should be gentle, especially if you are still

fragile or tired after the birth. Swimming, cycling or walking regularly are ideal. The jerky movements of jogging or skipping, though, have not been shown to improve the condition of cellulite.
● Dry skin brushing will also help. This is used by natural practitioners to help cleanse the body of unreleased toxins. It stimulates the circulation and lymphatic systems, encouraging the body's elimination systems to release wastes and thus breaking down determined fatty deposits.

Brushing the skin with a stiff dry brush – preferably natural bristle – will also encourage the removal of dead skin cells, unblock the pores and again help the body to eliminate wastes. It is invigorating and will make the skin glow, removing any dry, scaly skin. Done regularly, there will be a gradual reduction in cellulite and the legs and thighs will improve in tone and shape.

Dry skin brushing really needs to be done every day before a bath, preferably in the morning, as in the evening it will be too stimulating for the body and you may find you can't sleep afterwards.

Remember to brush very, very gently to begin with and that the number of times that you should brush, in the instructions below, are the ones you should work up to, not begin with. Always brush with long, firm strokes using a long-handled brush. If the brush is very scratchy at first, then soaking overnight to soften the bristles will help, and always remember to wash it frequently.

How to brush the skin

● Do one leg at a time, starting with the soles of the feet. Brush these and then brush over the foot, up to the knee and all around the leg. Do this about four times.
● Continue up the knee, along the thigh to the buttocks, where you can brush in circular movements and a little harder.
● Brush the arms starting at the hands and between each finger, working from the wrist to elbow and then up to the shoulder. To help the lymph glands under the arms, brush there in circular movements, five times one way, and then five times the other. Then brush the neck and back.
● Avoid the breasts, but brush the chest. Over the trunk and abdomen go a little more slowly and gently, working round the lower abdomen in a clockwise direction as this is the way the large bowel goes.

Note of caution: However beneficial skin brushing is, it is not a treatment I would recommend during the early days of lactation.

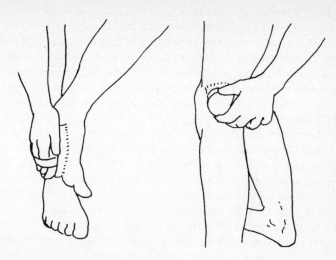

During this time, until your baby is at least eight weeks old, it would be better to cleanse the body with a gentle body scrub (see pages 94–95). This is because skin brushing is a very stimulating treatment and will encourage the body to leak milk.

Aromahelp

● I would recommend either a daily body scrub (in the first few months after the birth) or daily skin brushing (from at least two months after the birth) – see 94–95 above – followed by an essential oil bath and then perhaps a massage with essential oils:

Anti-cellulite bath

To a warm bath, add 2–3 drops of either rosemary, cypress or geranium oil. Swish the water to disperse the oil. Soak in the water for 10–15 minutes.

Anti-cellulite massage oil

To 50 ml (2½ tablespoons) of sweet almond oil or grapeseed oil, add 4 drops of geranium, 4 drops of cypress and 3 drops of rosemary oil. Mix well.

Use at least three times a week, after a bath.

● If you have very bad cellulite more than six months after the birth, it is worth visiting a qualified aromatherapist (see Appendix for how to find one in your area) who can help you to deal with it.

12

Post-baby
skin and hair

After the hormonal ups and downs of pregnancy and birth, the
condition of your skin can change temporarily. Even if it is
usually problem-free, it may become dry, oily or even prone to
spots. Essential oils can make a big difference to 'post-baby skin',
when part of a daily routine. The oils can penetrate through the
skin, sinking deep into the lower layers and getting to work on
the cells there before they start their journey to the skin's surface.
It takes three weeks for new, well-conditioned cells to reach the
top layer of skin (although as we age the process takes longer).
This explains why three weeks or so after being ill or run-down,
this can show in the condition of the skin. So if you have a special
date, book an aromatherapist three weeks in advance and be
vigilant about using essential oils for a daily massage (see Facial
Oils, page 100).

The condition of the hair can also change, sometimes
dramatically, during and after pregnancy. Normally bouncy and
problem-free hair can become dank and oily. Just as with the skin,
aromatherapy can help restore the condition of post-baby hair.

Post-baby skin

It would be foolish to expect any new (or not so new) mother to
perform an elaborate and time-consuming daily beauty ritual.
You will probably find that you have less time for yourself now
than you've ever had in your life – if this is your first baby this
can be something of a shock – so it's important if your skin is
suffering to find a simple routine that is easy to stick to. There is
no need to try all the suggestions that I make below. Just pick out

what appeals to you. The great bonus of essential oils is that not only can they be added to carrier oils, but they can be incorporated into any unperfumed creams or lotions you already use. Here are a few general tips:

● For the first three to four weeks after the baby is born, you will probably be too tired at night to do anything much more strenuous than have a quick wash or bath (don't forget to add essential oils to the water to help you relax and sleep, see page 57), but however tired you are, don't be tempted to get into bed without taking your make-up off – that is, if you've had time to put it on in the first place.

Cleanse your face and splash several times with tepid water to close the pores. Tone either with rose-water (available at the chemist) if your skin is dry to normal or orange flower water for oily to combination skin.

● After a bath or shower, continue to use Anti-Stretch Mark Oil (see pages 62–63). This will not only help to keep your skin soft and supple, but will help to prevent stretch marks that can form as your body shrinks back to its normal size. The orangey smell is also cheerfully uplifting.

Skin types

To get the best results, you should always use skin preparations that are suited to your particular type of skin. The following guidelines will help you to select from the various oils and creams that I give recipes for later in this chapter (see pages 100–103):

Dry or sensitive skin

This is fine – sometimes thin – skin that can react to harsh soaps or other beauty products. It needs protecting to help prevent the early appearance of dry lines.

Normal skin

This is neither dry nor oily and usually totally trouble-free, clear and unblemished.

Oily skin

Shiny, sallow and prone to open pores, this type of skin attracts grime and often suffers from spots and blackheads. The bonus is that it will remain youthful-looking the longest.

Combination skin

This is the name given to facial skin with a greasy central panel which like oily skin has a tendency to spots, blackheads and open pores. The rest of the face can be quite dry and sensitive, especially in those with red hair, so the skin needs balancing.

Allergic skin

This is very delicate fine skin that is prone to allergic reactions.

The condition of your skin will vary from time to time, especially during and after major changes in your life, such as pregnancy. So you may sometimes have to change the skin creams and lotions you use to match your current skin condition.

Facial oils

One of the best ways of caring for facial skin and treating any imbalances is a light facial massage. It has a soothing effect anyway, but the bonus is a dramatic improvement in the skin's condition.

Use one of the oils described below, according to your skin type. Note that for each skin type I have singled out essential oils that have proved to be especially popular and effective with my clients and which tie in with oils you will probably be familiar with from pregnancy. Certain oils appear under more than one skin type and this is because their balancing nature makes them suitable for many types of skin. The carrier oil I have used is jojoba – it is one I use and would particularly recommend as a facial oil – but almond or apricot oil can be substituted.

Dry or sensitive skin

To 10 ml (½ tablespoon) of jojoba oil (or almond or apricot), add 2 drops of either rose or sandalwood oil, or 1 drop of sandalwood and 1 drop of neroli oil, or 1 drop of sandalwood and 1 drop of rose oil.

Other suitable oils are Roman camomile, jasmine and ylang-ylang.

Normal skin

To 10 ml (½ tablespoon) of jojoba oil, add 2 drops of lavender or 2 drops of geranium oil, or 1 drop of neroli and 1 drop of lavender oil, or 1 drop of geranium and 1 drop of neroli oil.

Other suitable oils are sandalwood, rose and jasmine.

Oily skin

To 10 ml (½ tablespoon) of jojoba oil, add 2 drops of ylang-ylang or 2 drops of geranium oil, or 1 drop of lemon and 1 drop of lavender oil, or 1 drop of cypress and 1 drop of geranium oil.
Another suitable oil is sandalwood.

Combination skin

To 10 ml (½ tablespoon) of jojoba oil, add 2 drops of sandalwood or 2 drops of geranium oil, or 1 drop of geranium and 1 drop of ylang-ylang, or 1 drop of cypress and 1 drop of rose oil.
Other suitable oils are lavender and neroli.

Allergic skin

To 10 ml (½ tablespoon) of jojoba oil, add 1 drop of camomile and/or 1 drop of sandalwood oil.

• Facial oil can be used at any time, but leave an interval of at least one hour before putting make-up on – so probably the most practical time to apply is at night after cleansing the face, which also means the oil can sink into a restful skin.
• The massage doesn't have to be a lengthy job or done as in a beauty salon. Just stroke the oil into the face, neck and forehead with gentle, upward and circular movements. Avoid the eyes.
• Leave the oil on the face for at least ten minutes or as long as you can (a good time to do this is while relaxing in an essential oil bath). Then blot with a tissue to remove the residue oil before getting into bed. If your skin is very dry you may find all the oil has soaked in, but blot the skin anyway as any surplus may find its ways around the eyes during the night and can cause puffiness.
• Use 2–3 times a week, choosing an oil to suit your current skin condition. If you use oils to normalise an oily skin, monitor the skin's progress and change to different oils if the skin's condition changes.

Face creams

It is better to use creams on the face during the day; oils are better used at night.
Using the methods described below, try the following recipes for face creams, taking note of the following points:

• The essential oils I have singled out for each skin type are those that have proved to be popular and effective with my clients. The other oils recommended are also suitable to try.
• When buying unperfumed creams or lotions, make sure they don't contain lanolin as it can aggravate skin rashes.
• If the cream is in a plastic bottle, you will need to buy some glass jars (ask your pharmacist), as essential oils don't react well with plastic. Sterilise the jars before use – using sterilising fluid – and make sure they are dry by putting them in a low oven. Also sterilise a small thin-stemmed plastic utensil for mixing the creams, or boil a coffeespoon for five minutes to sterilise it.
• When making up the oils at home I suggest you stick to a 1 per cent dilution of the essential oils. For example:

A 1 per cent dilution of 50 g (2 oz) cream would contain 12 drops of essential oil.
A 1 per cent dilution of 30 g (1¼ oz) cream would contain 7 drops of essential oil.

• Following the directions for quantities, squeeze the cream into the jar and add the essential oils. Stir very well to make sure the oil is distributed evenly and don't forget to label the jar afterwards.

Dry or sensitive skin
To 30 g (1¼ oz) of cream base, add 3 drops of sandalwood, 3 drops of neroli and 1 drop of rose oil.
   Other suitable oils are Roman camomile, jasmine or ylang-ylang.

Normal skin
To 30 g (1¼ oz) of cream base, add 3 drops of neroli, 3 drops of sandalwood and 1 drop of jasmine oil.
   Other suitable oils are rose, lavender or geranium.

Oily skin
To 30 g (1¼ oz) of cream base, add 3 drops of lavender, 3 drops of geranium and 1 drop of lemon oil.
   Other suitable oils are sandalwood or ylang-ylang.

Combination skin
To 30 g (1¼ oz) of cream base, add 3 drops of geranium, 3 drops of rose and 1 drop of lavender oil.
   Other suitable oils are ylang-ylang and sandalwood.

Allergic skin

To 30 g (1¹/₄ oz) of cream base, add 2 drops of German camomile and 2 drops of sandalwood. You may increase the number of drops used up to 7 if the skin tolerates the cream well.

Another suitable oil is neroli.

Facial scrubs

Scrubs can be used on the face as well as on the body. If your skin is looking dingy or dull, a scrub will help to deep cleanse it by unclogging the pores and removing dirt and dead skin cells, leaving the skin fresh and glowing. It will then be more receptive to oils or creams.

Basic scrub mix

Mix together 100 g (4 oz) oatmeal and 100 g (4 oz) ground almonds. If you only have whole almonds, first remove the skins – make sure they are dry or they will go off when stored – and grind in a food processor.

Store the mixture in a glass jar and keep the lid on to keep dry.

Facial scrub

Place 1 teaspoonful of the Basic Scrub Mix (see above) in a basin. Add ¹/₂–1 teaspoon of jojoba, almond or apricot oil, or substitute the same amount of any of the following:

honey – for dry skin
yoghurt – for oily skin or blemishes
aloe gel – for irritated skin
rose-water – for sensitive skin or if you need a less abrasive scrub.

Add 1 drop of essential oil:

rose or sandalwood – for dry skin
rose, geranium, neroli or lavender – for normal skin
lavender, Roman camomile or lemon – for oily or blemish-prone skin
sandalwood, rose or Roman camomile – for sensitive skin
geranium or neroli – for combination skin.

Mix the blend together.

Apply to the face avoiding the under-eye area. Leave until the mixture feels dry (about 1–2 minutes), then rub off gently in small circular movements with damp fingers. Don't drag or stretch the skin. If your skin is very sensitive, you may prefer to rinse off the scrub, but it won't be so effective.

Post-baby hair

After pregnancy, the hair can be in quite poor shape and can become lank, greasy and even go to the other extreme and become very dry. Some women even discover that their normally curly hair becomes quite straight and vice versa. You may well notice an increase in hair loss. We all naturally lose between 80 and 100 hairs a day. But you may now notice even more. Don't panic, as this is extremely common after pregnancy and is a result of fluctuating hormone levels and possible nutritional deficiencies. Your hair will recover, but may need just a little help.

Here are a few tips:

● Eat a good, well-balanced diet with plenty of protein and Vitamin B. Avoid coffee and alcohol as they can deplete stores of B vitamins.
● Get a good haircut in a manageable style, preferably one that adds bounce and volume if your hair is lank.
● Gently massage your head when you wash your hair to encourage the blood supply to the scalp.

Aromahelp

Using essential oils can help to restore the condition of your hair. Try the following suggestions for pre-wash conditioners, hair rinses, shampoo and brushing.

Pre-wash conditioners
These will help the hair to become more manageable and shiny with a marked improvement in condition.

For dry or greasy hair and to help stimulate the scalp if there is hair loss, add 10 drops of rosemary and 10 drops of lavender oil to 60 ml (3 tablespoons) of almond oil and 40 ml (2 tablespoons) of jojoba oil.

For any dry hair condition or dandruff, add 10 drops of tea-tree and 10 drops of lavender oil to 60 ml (3 tablespoons) of almond oil and 40 ml (2 tablespoons) of jojoba oil.

Pour about 20 ml (1 tablespoon) of the mixture into a small bowl. Using the fingertips, massage the oil gently into the scalp.

Wrap the hair in a towel and leave for at least one hour before washing the hair.

Use this treatment at least twice weekly if your hair is in bad condition.

Hair rinses

As a child my mother used to rinse my hair in water and cider vinegar to keep it 'squeaky clean and shiny'. Cider vinegar does actually help to restore the acid mantle – the protective barrier that is removed with alkaline shampoos. It is also very helpful for itchy scalps or dandruff.

To 300 ml (½ pint) of warm water, add 30 ml (1½ tablespoons) of cider vinegar.

Add 2 drops of the recommended essential oils below:

sandalwood, lavender, rosemary, geranium or Roman camomile – for dry or normal hair
lemon, cypress, lavender or rosemary – for oily hair
tea-tree, lavender, sandalwood, cypress or rosemary – for a dry scalp or dandruff
tea-tree, Roman camomile, rosemary, lemon or lavender – for thinning hair
rose or jasmine – for an indulgent treat.

Use as a final rinse (i.e. don't rinse it out), working well into the hair.

Shampoo

To about 10 ml (½ tablespoon) of very mild baby shampoo, add 1 drop of any of the essential oils recommended for the hair rinse above (select the oil according to hair type) and stir well.

Wash as normal (pouring shampoo on to hair before adding water can make it easier to wash).

Fragrant brushing

To help stimulate the circulation on the scalp, put 1 drop of rosemary oil on a hairbrush. Bend your head forwards and brush the hair downwards towards the floor.

13
Baby massage

Some of the most enjoyable times for you and your baby can come through the closeness of a cuddle at feeding time, whether you breast- or bottle-feed. Touch is very important for tiny babies. Touch given and received by the parents helps the bonding process and this is where aromatherapy massage can help. Massage for babies can be just as valuable as massage for adults.

Research from round the world has confirmed that babies who are massaged regularly feed and sleep better than those who aren't, and that colic and constipation are reduced. The London obstetrician Yehudi Gordon is very enthusiastic about baby massage and agrees that 'massage helps parents communicate with their baby, thereby strengthening the bonding process'.

This early bonding is especially important for the mothers of premature babies. In 1988, a research report from the USA showed the great effectiveness of early infant-mother stimulation through talking, rocking, eye contact and massage. New research from The Touch Research Institute at the University of Miami School shows that massage also plays an important role in physical development, proving that it can have major health advantages. It appears that massage encourages more efficient absorption of food (premature babies gained on average 47 per cent more weight per day than those who did not receive massage) and that massaged babies were more responsive, active and alert and suffered less anxiety.

Baby massage oil

The following formula is perfect to use as a general massage oil when your baby is happy, though it will also help to calm and relax him when he is not. It will help keep his skin free from the bacteria that cause nappy rash and will leave his skin clean and sweet smelling. Use it instead of the mineral-based baby oils, which, although they are good at keeping the baby 'water-proofed', are not ideal as massage oil as they clog the pores.

It is useful to make up a 100 ml bottle as it saves time to always have a massage oil ready to hand. Keep it somewhere cool with the cap screwed tightly on and always away from other children.

Aromatic baby massage oil

To 100 ml (5 tablespoons) of almond oil or 80 ml (4 tablespoons) of almond oil and 20 ml (1 tablespoon) of jojoba oil, add 2 drops of Roman camomile, rose, neroli or lavender oil, or 1 drop of rose and 1 drop of Roman camomile oil.

If you prefer a smaller quantity, just use 50 ml (2½ tablespoons) of almond oil or 30 ml (1½ tablespoons) of almond oil and 20 ml (1 tablespoon) of jojoba, and add just 1 drop of rose, Roman camomile, lavender or neroli oil.

For babies that have colic or other tummy troubles, the following oil is helpful:

Colic baby massage oil

To 100 ml (5 tablespoons) of almond oil or 80 ml (4 tablespoons) of almond oil and 20 ml (1 tablespoon) of jojoba oil, add 2 drops of tangerine, mandarin or camomile oil.

If you prefer a smaller quantity, just use 50 ml (2½ tablespoons) of almond oil, or 30 ml (1½ tablespoons) of almond oil and 20 ml (1 tablespoon) of jojoba, and add just 1 drop of tangerine, mandarin or camomile oil.

Babies and young children should always have very low amounts of essential oils. Never be tempted to use more – the amounts given above are the maximum I would recommend for babies under one year. As with homeopathic remedies, less is better than more.

Tips for massaging your baby

● When the time is right, give your baby a massage. Choose a time when he is content (perhaps after a bath or nappy-free playtime). Don't attempt to massage him if he is tired, hungry or fretful, although once you are both used to massaging him, you may find he can be comforted by it (such as a tummy or lower-back rub for colic).

● It is important that you aren't tired or in a hurry, or your baby will sense your mood and the experience of massage will not be as happy as it should be.

● Have everything that you need ready before you begin – towel, oil, clean nappy, and clothes.
● Make sure the room is warm.
● You should have short nails and remove any jewellery to avoid scratching the baby.
● Don't massage for longer than 10 minutes or your baby will get bored.
● If your baby doesn't enjoy the massage, stop at once and try again another time.
● When your baby is facing you, keep eye contact with him. Smile or talk and let him know this is something to feel happy about.
● The safest way to massage your baby is to sit on the floor with your legs outstretched, a large towel placed over your lap and the baby on top. If you find that difficult, then try putting him on a large towel in the middle of the bed, but don't ever leave him alone like this – even the smallest of babies can somehow manage to wriggle to the edge.
● If the phone rings in the middle of the massage, take your baby with you, remembering to wrap him in a towel and wipe your hands, otherwise you may have an oily baby slipping right out of your arms.
● You don't need to be a practised masseuse. Just do what you think feels good for your baby. Massage gently and lovingly, building to a gentle rhythm. Always massage upwards, towards the heart.
● Most important of all, talk to him reassuringly throughout the massage, or sing to him and generally make it an enjoyable experience for both of you.

How to massage your baby

You will soon find your own routine but this may help to begin with:

● Start by lying your baby on his back – he can then see what you are doing.
● Using both hands – one on either leg – start from the ankles and massage a small amount of oil up to the tops of the legs. Then glide your hands down again to the feet. There should never be any pressure in the downward glide in either adult or baby massage, as this goes against the flow of the circulation. Repeat three or four times.

● Take each foot with all of your fingers. Support the front of the foot and massage the sole in circular movements with your thumbs, first in one direction, then the other. Repeat three or four times. This is a very calming movement for your baby and one you may find yourself returning to again and again when he needs comforting, such as during a bout of crying.

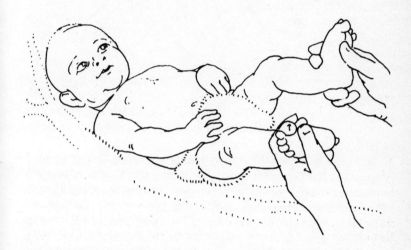

● From the feet stroke your hands up the legs to the abdomen and using the palm of one hand gently massage the abdomen in a clockwise direction. This is a very useful movement when your baby has colic or is constipated.
● Move up to and circle around the shoulders. Glide gently down the arms to the wrists and up to the shoulders again. Repeat three to four times.
● If your baby is still quite happy, turn him over with his head facing your feet, making sure his head isn't squashed, or lie him across your lap (obviously in this position you can only use one hand for massage).
● Massage the back of the legs from ankles to bottom. Place your hands on the top of the buttocks and glide them with one hand on either side of the spine (unless he is lying across your lap, in which case just use one hand and keep the other free to secure him) up to the neck and out over the shoulders and back down the sides of the body to the buttocks again. Repeat.

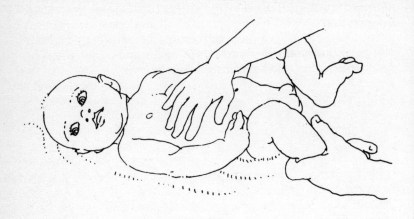

Note: Don't massage the baby's hands as there is a risk he may pass oil from these to his mouth or eyes. I also think it's best not to massage the face as again oil can get into eyes and mouth. Also, some babies don't like large hands coming down on their face and there is always a chance you could stick a finger in the baby's eye.

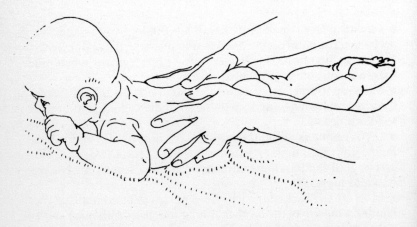

14

Aromahelp for baby problems

Essential oils, with their gentle, calming and healing properties, can help your baby when he is overtired or not feeling well. They can also help to keep the nursery smelling sweet and fresh. If your baby can't be comforted by the means discussed in this chapter or seems at all ill, then your first call should be to your doctor. Babies can become ill surprisingly quickly. Don't worry about being a nuisance to the doctor – in 18 years of being a doctor's wife, I have never heard my husband complain when an anxious mother has rung him, even at three in the morning.

Seek immediate medical help if your baby or child has any of the following:

- Fever (38°C *and above*)
- Unexplained drowsiness
- Severe headaches
- Convulsions or fits
- Altered responsiveness and/or irritability
- Severe vomiting and/or diarrhoea
- Dislike of light
- Refusing feeds
- Obvious pain and distress

Baby snuffles

Having a cold must be very frustrating if you are a baby, as you can't blow your nose. Some babies get the snuffles even without having a cold and find it difficult to breathe when sleeping or feeding.

Aromahelp

● Using essential oils in a vaporiser in your baby's room or the room where you feed him will help to kill airborne bacteria, freshen the air and help him to breathe a little easier. A vaporiser can be used and then removed before your baby goes into the room.

To a vaporiser or bowl of hot water, add 2–4 drops of lemon, eucalyptus, lavender or tea-tree oil.

Bumps and bruises

Apply an essential oil cold compress as soon as possible to reduce swelling and bruising.

Aromahelp

● Add 2–3 drops of lavender to 300 ml (½ pint) of cold water. Agitate the water to mix the drops. Lay a cloth or clean flannel on top of water to pick up the oils. Squeeze out excess water and lay the cloth on the bruised area. Repeat as necessary. *Do not massage any swelling*.

Constipation

Persistent constipation or constipation with obvious distress and pain needs medical treatment.

● In the absence of medical problems intermittent constipation in young babies can be due to lack of fluids. Give frequent drinks of water or diluted fruit juice. Older babies and toddlers will benefit from more soluble fibre in their diet. This can be found in porridge oats, apples, bananas and, carrots. *Do not give bran.*

Toddlers can become anxious during toilet training and will 'hang on', not opening their bowels for several days. This can mean passing painful motions, which in turn leads to them holding back again. Keep a relaxed attitude and let your child see that bowel function is individual and normal.

Aromahelp

If your baby is prone to passing infrequent hard stools encourage bowel movement with gentle massage.

Use a little of the following blend and massage the lower abdomen and lower back in a clockwise action twice a day for three to four days (see also Chapter 13: Baby Massage):

Constipation massage oil
● Add 1 drop of Roman camomile and 1 drop of mandarin to 20 ml (1 tablespoon) of carrier oil. Use a little of this blend twice a day.
● A warm bath with 1–2 drops of lavender diluted in 1 tablespoon of full-fat milk can help ease any pain. If your toddler is expressing anxiety and is frightened of opening his bowels give a warm, comforting lavender bath, whatever the time of day.

Cradle cap

Cradle cap is very common in new-born or small babies. There are flaky patches on the scalp which come off in large pieces. The scalp is often greasy.

Aromahelp

● Massage the scalp with Aromatic Baby Massage Oil (see page 107), which has already been blended with an equal amount of jojoba oil. Massage about a teaspoon into the scalp – not just the hair – very, very gently once or twice a day.
● Also try this shampoo:

Cradle cap shampoo
To a normal 50 ml size of baby shampoo, add 1–2 drops of tea-tree oil and mix well.

Always shake well before using and only apply a small amount.

Avoid the eyes and rinse well after shampooing.

Use daily for one week or until the scalp looks clearer. Then use occasionally as the need arises.

Diarrhoea

Severe diarrhoea with or without vomiting in young babies always needs medical treatment. Babies can quickly become dehydrated and very ill.

If your child is not too unwell, a warm bath or gentle tummy massage with essential oils can be comforting and help relieve cramping pains.

Aromatic bath

Add 1–2 drops of camomile, sandalwood or lavender diluted in full-fat milk to a warm bath.

Massage

Add 1–2 drops of camomile to 50 ml (2½ tablespoons) of carrier oil. Massage a little of the oil into baby's tummy. *Don't massage if your baby has recently vomited, or you think he is feeling sick.*

Eczema

I am often asked if there are any essential oils that will ease eczema. There are, but I feel it is better to take the child to a qualified aromatherapist for expert advice and to let her see the condition of the skin. She will then make up the correct oils.

Infantile colic

Sometimes otherwise healthy babies of between six and 14 weeks wail for long periods every night and can't be comforted by anything. They are not thirsty, they don't *appear* to have wind or feel sick and even a clean nappy and a cuddle fails to comfort them. The crying usually follows a set time pattern – in fact you could almost set your watch by it. It is usually in the early evening. The baby may stop for a brief time while being rocked, but this is short-lived. This pattern of crying may be what is called 'evening crying'. Here there is no physical cause. Some babies just cry and are miserable and inconsolable, which is very distressing, especially for a first-time mother who probably feels insecure enough about her mothering skills without her baby seeming to complain so vocally.

In some cases, however, there is a physical reason for this regular pattern of crying – infantile or 'three-month' colic. Here the baby does have wind and is in pain, although it is often difficult to tell, so it is best if your baby cries regularly to assume that he might have colic and to take appropriate action.

In Europe, massage is widely used for the treatment of colic. In 1989, from his practice in Denmark, Dr Jan-Helge Larson demonstrated the success of both belly massage – carried out over the clothes without oil – and whole body massage with oil. He also established that there can be several causes of colic, which range from insufficient winding to the parent's insecurity being transmitted to the baby. At his clinic, parents were shown how to massage as well as how to wind and correctly position the baby for feeding. He also demonstrated that parents need support and understanding during this difficult time.

Here are some tips that may help you if you have a baby who cries regularly and who may be suffering from colic:

● Try giving him a belly massage. There is no need to undress him for this massage. Sit down, with plenty of room on either side of your elbows, and hold the baby in your lap with his tummy downwards and his body sticking up a little. With one hand, massage his abdomen, starting in the middle at his navel and then gently working around in larger and larger circles in a clockwise direction. Dr Larson (see above) recommends doing this massage 15–30 minutes after a feed.

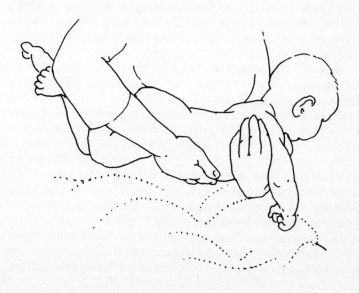

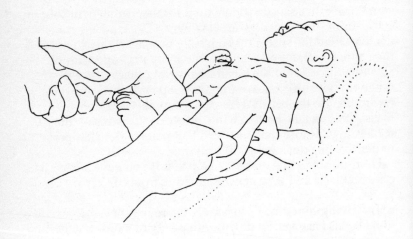

● Keep calm – he may bawl his head off when you are starting any of these remedies but hopefully he will stop as you get them underway.

● Take his nappy off and by very gently bending one or both knees up towards his tummy and making cycling movements, you can help to establish if he has trapped wind or is having trouble opening his bowels. Only do this movement a few times.

● After a feed, allow sufficient time for him to bring his wind up before laying him down. Not even adults can burp to order. Even if he doesn't ever have sicky burps never lie him down on his back as he could choke. Always lie him on his side.

● Movement can help, so try putting him in his pram and pushing it backwards and forwards (I've done this in the past with my foot whilst peeling potatoes at the kitchen sink) or park the pram next to a switched-on tumble dryer, as the noise can be comforting.

● Sometimes foods that are passed on through breast-milk can upset a baby, particularly spicy foods such as curry and wind-producing foods such as sprouts, so check your diet and see if there is any connection with his crying.

● If you are bottle-feeding ask your health visitor for advice.

● Not all babies suffer from colic; some small babies cry because they are hungry or thirsty, so try feeding or offer some cooled boiled water.

• Don't worry about 'spoiling' your baby by picking him up to comfort him. You can't spoil a tiny baby – he is not aware enough to manipulate you – and if he is crying it is because he is trying to tell you something is upsetting him. If a cuddle soothes him, don't feel guilty about giving him what he needs.

• It may sound easy to say now, but rest assured that this awful time will end – usually, it seems, at around three months. Sometimes the only thing to do is to adapt your life around it, by preparing meals before the expected crying time, planning anything important in the evening around it. Try not to see this as the baby ruling you, more a few measures for self-preservation. If you have gone back to work, don't blame yourself. Babies still cry for hours on end when their mothers stay at home.

Aromahelp

• Undress your baby, lie him on a warm towel and massage his lower back. Then turn him over and massage his abdomen in a gentle clockwise movement. This will help dispel wind. Let him suckle at your breast after his massage. Hopefully he will go to sleep in your arm and you can then put him straight to bed.

This massage can be done without oil or you can use the ready-made-up Aromatic Baby Massage Oil (see page 107) or the following:

Roman camomile baby oil
Add 2 drops of Roman camomile oil to 100 ml (5 tablespoons) of almond oil. Mix well.

• Give your baby a warm bath.

For babies of three months or over, add just 1 drop of Roman camomile oil to 20 ml (1 tablespoon) milk. Agitate well, then pour this mixture into the warm bath water. Never put essential oils neat into a baby's bath water. If the oil doesn't disperse properly it can get into the baby's eyes. Also never use essential oils in a bath for a baby under three months old.

• Calm your baby down by scenting his room.

To a diffuser or on a cotton-wool ball placed near a radiator, add 1–2 drops of neroli. If you have other young children put the cotton-wool ball well out of their reach just in case they throw it into the baby's cot.

• Looking after a crying baby can be exhausting. If you become too upset or tired, ask someone in the house to look after your baby for a short time while you leave the room. Then try and relax for a few minutes.

An inhalation may help to calm you. On a tissue or clean handkerchief, put 1 drop of any of the following essential oils and sniff: petitgrain, geranium, mandarin, rose, bergamot, ylang-ylang, lemon, lavender, rosemary or grapefruit.

● When your baby has calmed down, run yourself a warm bath. Add 4–5 drops of any of the following oils to the water: petitgrain, geranium, mandarin, rose, bergamot, ylang-ylang, lemon, lavender, rosemary or grapefruit.

Minor burns/scalds

Seek immediate medical treatment for anything but minor burns and scalds.

Aromahelp

Lavender's soothing properties can quickly take the sting out of burns and will help calm any distress.

Babies under 1 year

● Add 2 drops of lavender to a bowl of very cold water and use a small cloth as a compress to lay over the burnt area. Repeat several times. If you like, you can add a little aloe vera gel to the lavender. *Do not apply this to babies' fingers as they might ingest the gel.*

Babies over 1 year

● If the burn is accessible, hold the burnt area under cold water for as long as you can. *It is recommended that burnt areas be held for at least ten minutes under cold water. Being realistic this is sometimes impossible with a young child.* Make up a solution of 2 drops of lavender to a bowl of very cold water. Lay a cloth on the water and apply to the burn as a compress. If you like, smear a little Aloe Gel with Lavender onto the burn:

Aloe gel with lavender

*For minor burns and sunbur*n. Add 2 drops of lavender to 10 ml (1/2 tablespoon) of aloe gel.

Minor wounds

Cuts and scratches

Essential oils of tea-tree and lavender have antiseptic, antibiotic and anti-fungal actions.

Aromahelp

Wash and clean minor wounds with a tepid solution of 2–3 drops of lavender or tea-tree essential oils diluted in 300 ml (½ pint) water.

If needed use a little Healing gel and/or cover with gauze or a plaster.

Healing gel

Add 6 drops of lavender and 6 drops of tea-tree to a 50 g (2 oz) jar of aloe gel. Mix well. Keep the pot in a cool place ready for family first aid.

Nappy rash

All babies get a sore bottom from time to time, but consult your doctor if the rash won't clear up.

Here are some tips to help:

- If your baby develops nappy rash, change nappies frequently. Never leave him in a wet nappy, especially a soiled one. Let him have as much nappy-free time as possible, as sore and chapped skin needs the air.
- Try to keep your baby's bottom dry as much as possible.
- If you are using terry nappies, ensure they are well rinsed and free from any trace of washing powder or chemical cleaner.
- Wipe your baby's bottom clean with damp cotton-wool or jojoba oil (which is particularly good). Anything dry will drag and irritate sore places.

Aromahelp

Use some Roman camomile Baby Oil (see page 117) sparingly at nappy change.

Apply the following cream to ease soreness and fight the bacteria that causes nappy rash:

Nappy rash cream

To a 50 g (2 oz) pot if unperfumed cream (one that doesn't contain lanolin), add 2 drops of German camomile and 2 drops of lavender oil, or if you health visitor thinks that the rash may be caused by thrush, add 4 drops of tea-tree oil instead.

Use this cream very sparingly a couple of times a day (depending on the soreness of the bottom). To be extra safe, try on a small test area first, as babies' skins vary and some sore bottoms should just be kept clean, dry and well aired.

● For babies over 3 months with nappy rash, try this bath:

Nappy rash bath

To 20 ml (1 tablespoon) of full-fat milk, add 1 drop of lavender or 1 drop of Roman camomile oil. Agitate well and add to a warm bath.

For babies over six months with nappy rash, 1 drop of tea-tree oil can be substituted for the lavender or Roman camomile oil above.

● If you are using terry or cloth nappies, try soaking them before washing in a bucket of water (having first removed any solid matter) to which you have added 6–8 drops of either lavender or tea-tree essential oil or 3 drops of lavender and 3 drops of tea-tree oil (this smells nicer). Leave for 2–3 hours before washing in the normal way. This will help disinfect the nappies.

You can also add lavender oil to the final rinse after washing. If rinsing by hand, add 1–2 drops of oil to a large bowl of water. When using a washing machine, add 4–5 drops along with the fabric conditioner.

Sunburn

If your child has severe sunburn or shows signs of being unwell, you should seek professional medical help. Babies and little children quickly become ill and dehydrated if they have too much sun.

● Cool and soothe any burnt areas as quickly as possible.
● Keep the child cool and quiet, and give plenty of fluids.
● As with other burns, a lavender essential oil compress laid on the skin can help take the redness and sting away (see compress under Minor Burns/Scalds above).

• Apply plain aloe vera juice well diluted in water liberally to the skin.
• Put the child into a tepid bath with 2 drops of lavender oil. *In this instance it is best not to dilute the oils in milk first.* Gently pat the child dry to avoid dragging the skin, dress in loose clothes and keep cool. Repeat the bath after two hours if necessary.
• Make up a fine spray-mist bottle containing 300 ml (½ pint) of cold water and 2 drops of lavender oil. Shake the bottle very well to mix the oils. Use the mix to spray burnt unbroken skin on the back, trunk, legs and arms. *Do not use on the face or fingers, or on very young babies.*

Teething

There is no set age when teething begins – some babies can be born with teeth and with others the first won't emerge until they are 12 months old. However, in general most babies cut their first tooth at around five to six months, when you may notice a number of symptoms. You may find your baby becoming irritable or fretful, dribbling a lot, chewing on anything he can get hold of but especially his fists and hands, scratching his ears and he may even develop flushed cheeks. Take care, though, not to blame other symptoms on teething – if your baby is feverish, or suffers from vomiting, diarrhoea, or lack of appetite, see your doctor.

If your baby is teething, offer him something hard to chew on, e.g. a cooled teething ring or a rusk. Rubbing his gums with a cool, clean finger can also help.

Aromahelp

• To a vaporiser or bowl of hot water, add 1–2 drops of Roman camomile or lavender oil. Place this in your baby's room.
• Use this massage oil, but only on babies of six months or over:

Massage oil for teething

To 100 ml (5 tablespoons) of sweet almond oil, add 1 drop of lavender and 1 drop of Roman camomile oil. Mix well.

Rub just a smear (no more than 2 drops) along the jawline to the ear of a teething baby. Do *not* rub on the upper cheekbone near the eye or near the mouth.

Wakeful and restless toddlers

Older babies and young children fail to settle at night for a wide variety of reasons. They could be hungry, thirsty, frightened of the dark (especially if older children tease them with bogeymen stories), frightened that you might not come back or it could simply be that life downstairs sounds just too exciting to miss. Some children become quite hyperactive at bedtime and all efforts to stop them climbing out of their cot fail.

If your child is not tired, let him come downstairs for a while and tire himself out. That way everyone is happy. There is little comfort for anyone letting a miserable child stay upstairs. But this can become a habit that is difficult to break, so try to establish a bedtime routine, which can be quite comforting for even small babies.

Children and babies always seem to instinctively know when their parents are going out and have difficulty settling when they sense it, so try not to hurry bedtime on those occasions and get them ready for bed well before you leave the house.

Aromahelp

● Most children do unwind with a warm bath. I don't recommend using essential oils in the bath for babies under three months old, but after that age they can be very helpful. Do use discretion, though, with small babies that get distressed every night. They obviously cry for very different reasons than toddlers do and, for them, aromatherapy baths are not recommended on a regular basis.

Calming bath

To a cup or bowl containing 10–20 ml (½–1 tablespoon) of full-fat milk, add 1–2 drops of Roman camomile oil. Stir well and add to the warm bath. Then mix well in the water.

My advice to mothers who are having trouble getting their children to sleep is to give this Roman camomile bath every other night for a week, then for two or three nights the following week. At the end of a fortnight, hopefully the child will have got back into a regular sleep pattern again.

Roman camomile oil, though very mild and suitable for children, is best not used continuously but just when needed, so a child should not be given a camomile bath as a matter of course.

A word of caution

Some people use essential oils on a baby's bedding and clothing. I wouldn't recommend doing this, as the neat oils could come into contact with the baby's skin.

Also, if using cotton-wool balls perfumed with essential oils to scent a baby's room never put them directly into the baby's cot and do take care with the amount of essential oil used (whether you use cotton-wool or a vaporiser). For babies of under a year old use only 1–2 drops and no more. For babies over a year old, this can be increased to 3–4 drops.

15

Preconceptual care

I am often asked by clients what I feel about preconceptual care and my reply is always the same: it takes two to make a baby. This means a prospective mother should only welcome top-quality sperm for top-quality eggs and time should be spent getting your body as healthy as possible so this can be achieved.

In the real world, some of us won't have the chance to plan a baby, as they have the habit of arriving at the most unexpected times. But if you are starting with a clean sheet, my advice is that a pre-birth plan should start six months before conception. Obviously, the longer you spend on this plan the better, but if you are in a hurry then three months will do. Any couple wishing to plan a baby should individually take responsibilitiy for the care of their own bodies.

The general plan involves basic common sense:

- Stop smoking and avoid any unnecessary drugs.
- Avoid any known pollutants or chemicals.
- Eat a well-balanced and healthy diet (plenty of vegetables, fruit, protein, etc.) and increase your intake of foods rich in zinc and B vitamins.
- Cut down on stimulants such as tea, coffee and alcohol (too much alcohol can have an effect on sperm production). Also avoid too much fat or sugar in your diet.
- Watch your weight and try to keep it neither under nor over what it should be. Take plenty of exercise to keep the body well toned and supple. Get plenty of rest.
- Stop using oral contraceptives.
- If you have any health problems or worries about genetically inheritied diseases, see your doctor, and if you suffer from minor or stress-related health problems, see an aromatherapist.

Failure to conceive

Any couple trying, but failing, to conceive should obviously see their doctor. However, it is still a good idea to put all the general guidelines given above for preconceptual care into action to give yourselves the best possible chance of conceiving.

Many couples who have been told there are no medical reasons for failing to conceive still fail to do so, which causes not only increasing levels of disappointment but also guilt, resentment and tension – all of which can ruin or destroy your sex life. This is where aromatherapy can help. I see many women in my treatment rooms who may come to me for other reasons, but who mention their anxiety over failure to conceive.

I am in no way suggesting the following are fertility formulas, but they can greatly reduce the tension between a couple in these difficult circumstances. So why not try them, along with the general preconceptual care.

Aromahelp

● These are the oils I use to help people with problems conceiving:

Rose (either Rosa centifolia *or* Rosa damascena)

Known as the perfect skin oil, rose is also described as a uterine tonic, as it is cleansing and regulating for the uterus. I find it helpful for clients with premenstrual tension or painful, heavy periods. It is also a good tension reliever and is reputed to have aphrodisiac qualities. Although a very feminine oil, it is thought to increase semen production, so is useful in a massage or bath blend for both partners.

Geranium

Geranium is an aromatic oil with many properties, including having a tonic action on the entire body and a hormonal balancing effect on the reproductive system. It is an excellent oil for any condition where anxiety and stress may be a factor ... and it smells lovely too!

Sandalwood

This oil has a heavy lingering aroma and is highly prized for its effect on male impotence. It is a highly relaxing oil and works well where depression has led to sexual problems or when there is anxiety.

Ylang-ylang

An exotically scented oil frequently used in relxing massage and bath blends, it gives a pleasantly romantic smell to the skin. It is used in cases of nervous tension, anxiety and impotence.

● Use the following oils for a relaxing massage, paying special attention to the lower back, abdomen, groin and hip area. Don't use the oils directly on the delicate genital area, as they could sting:

Massage oil for her

Add 15 drops of geranium and 5 drops of rose oil to 50 ml (2½ tablespoons) of almond oil. Mix well.

Massage oil for him

Add 5 drops of clary sage and 5 drops of rose, 5 drops of geranium and 5 drops of either sandalwood or ylang-ylang oil to 50 ml (2½ tablespoons) of almond oil. Mix well.

● Try the following bath mixes:

Blend 1 is relaxing and can be used by both of you during the evening.
   To a warm, full bath, add 4 drops of geranium, 2 drops of rose and 2 drops of clary sage oil. Swish the water to disperse the oil. Relax and soak for 10–15 minutes.

Blend 2 is for women to use as a morning bath.
   To a full bath, add 4 drops of geranium and 2 drops of rose oil. Swish the water to disperse the oil. Soak for 10 minutes.

   These baths can be enjoyed up to four times a week.

Aim to have a least two baths and two massages each per week whilst on this programme. Good luck!

16

A reference guide to essential oils

There are many essential oils available on the market, but in this chapter I have only listed the oils that are mentioned throughout the book. These are the oils I have used successfully on my clients and can recommend personally.

A–Z of essential oils

This is a guide to some, but not all, of the properties and general uses of essential oils. But remember that unless you are really familiar with essential oils, it is best, especially during pregnancy and for young children, to only use them as directly in the recipes and instructions for baths, oils, creams and gels, etc. given in this book.

Benzoin *(Styrax benzoin)*

Part of plant used   Gum resin exuded from the trunk of benzoin tree.
Where produced   Thailand; Malaysia; East Indies.
Aroma   Warm, vanilla smell.
Price band   Middle.
Main properties and effects   Antiseptic; diuretic; expectorant; healing; sedative.
Main uses   Benzoin is a pulmonary antiseptic and can be used as an inhalation to help expel mucus and relieve respiratory congestion. When used in a postnatal massage, it creates a feeling of warmth and comfort for those feeling emotionally cold. It is helpful for those with poor circulation and stiff, cold joints. It helps heal dry, cracked skin and sores and blends well with lemon

oil in a cream for rough, cracked hands. Use postnatally in a cream or gel for cracked and sore nipples.

It is thick and will be slow to pour from the bottle. It will solidify when kept under cold conditions, but will thin readily when brought to room temperature. It keeps well.

Ways to use   Inhalations; body massage; skin care.
Preconceptual care   No.
Pregnancy   No.
Labour   No.
Postnatally   Yes.
Babies   No.

Bergamot *(Citrus bergamia)*

Part of plant used   Expressed from the rind of the fruit.
Where produced   Southern Italy; North-west Africa.
Aroma   Fresh; citrus; sweet-smelling.
Price band   Middle.
Main properties and effects   Analgesic; antiseptic; anti-depressant; anti-spasmodic; anti-viral; deodorant; healing; refreshing; uplifting.
Main uses   Bergamot is the oil used to scent and flavour Earl Grey tea. It is very uplifting when feeling depressed or physically or mentally fatigued. It is indicated for some types of eczema and for skin conditions that have been brought on by stress. Use well diluted, alone or with lavender, to help infected spots, boils and wounds. It is one of the best oils to help relieve urinary and genital infections, particularly for those prone to frequent attacks of cystitis. Used as a bath oil during feverish illness (colds, flu, etc.) bergamot is cooling. It makes an ideal bath oil to help ward off depression during convalescence.
Ways to use   Body massage; facial oil; skin care; vaporisation; baths; showers; local application; compresses.
Preconceptual care   No.
Pregnancy   Yes (in room fresheners and sparingly for cystitis).
Labour   No.
Postnatally   Yes.
Babies   No.

Caution: Bergamot must not be used before sunbathing or going on a sun bed as it can cause uneven pigmentation.

Camomile, Roman *(Anthemis nobilis)* and German *(Matricaria chamomilla)*

Part of plant used   Distilled from the dried flowers.
Where produced   Italy.
Aroma   Pungent dried grass/herby smell.
Price band   Middle to expensive.
Main properties and effects   Antiseptic; analgesic; anti-inflammatory; anti-spasmodic.
Main uses   Like lavender, this oil is a first-aid kit in a bottle. Its aroma is either liked or loathed. It contains an anti-inflammatory substance called azulene, which gives it its familiar blue colour. Roman camomile can, however, vary from pale watery blue to colourless. German camomile has a thicker consistency and contains a higher proportion of azulene. It should be a deep blue, but tends to turn greenish yellow-brown as it ages or after frequent exposure to the air. German camomile also tends to be expensive. Do not confuse these two camomiles with camomile maroc, which is not from the same family (always check that your suppliers' list gives the Latin name of essential oils).

Its action helps calm, soothe and control many skin problems and allergies. Its anti-inflammatory and pain-relieving actions help soothe dull nagging pain, e.g. muscular aches, toothache, teething pain, headaches, chronic orthopaedic problems. Its anti-spasmodic action is excellent for period pains, indigestion, flatulence and especially babies' colic.

Camomile is a gentle sedative for young and old. It relaxes those who are stressed, anxious, irritable or having trouble sleeping and can help calm overtired or fretful children before bed.

Ways to use   Body massage; facial oil; skin care; baths; showers; local application; compresses; vaporisation.
Preconceptual care   No.
Pregnancy   Yes.
Labour   No.
Postnatally   Yes.
Babies   Yes.

Clary Sage *(Salvia sclarea)*

Part of plant used   Distilled from whole plant.
Where produced   Europe.
Aroma   Sweetish; nutty; exotic; heavy.
Price band   Middle.

Main properties and effects   Antiseptic; anti-depressant; anti-spasmodic; emmenagogue; aphrodisiac; uterine tonic.

Main uses   Used in aromatherapy in preference to common sage, which is very strong and can be toxic even in small doses. Clary sage is non-toxic, but should still be used in small quantities – a 1 per cent dilution is ideal. If used in too high a quantity it can be euphoric, leaving one feeling light-headed. It should not be used in treatment before driving a car or before drinking alcohol. Although suitable for both sexes, I think of clary sage essentially as a feminine oil. It helps regulate hormonal imbalance (it contains natural plant hormones resembling oestrogen). It is helpful for premenstrual tension and strongly indicated for menopausal symptoms. It can help lower high blood pressure. Its anti-depressant action makes it one of the best oils I know for postnatal blues. During labour it can be used as a compress to help relieve pain. Reputedly an aphrodisiac, its aroma is sensual and its relaxing, anti-depressant and euphoric actions do seem to help dispel any tension a couple may be experiencing.

Ways to use   Body massage; facial oil; baths; showers; vaporisation; compresses.

Preconceptual care   Yes.

Pregnancy   No.

Labour   Yes.

Postnatally   Yes.

Babies   No.

Cypress *(Cupressus sempervirens)*

Part of plant used   Distilled from the needles, cones and twigs of the tree.

Where produced   Europe.

Aroma   Woody; spicy; medicinal.

Price band   Middle.

Main properties and effects   Antiseptic; anti-spasmodic; astringent; deodorant; diuretic.

Main uses   It is used for problems associated with a sluggish, poor circulation, such as fluid retention, cramp, thread veins, varicose veins and ulcers. Its locally constricting action on capillaries makes it invaluable for treating haemorrhoids. Its powerful astringent action is similar to that of witch hazel. Postnatally it helps heal over sore perineal areas.

Its properties can help control excessive amounts of body fluid, such as in menorrhagia (heavy periods). Its suits oily and combination skin. As a bath oil is has a deodorant effect, helps to reduce perspiration and is relaxing and refreshing. It has a gentle sedative action on nervous tension. Its anti-spasmodic action will help relieve coughing.

Ways to use   Body massage; skin care; local application; compresses; baths; showers; vaporisation.

Preconceptual care   No.

Pregnancy   Yes (after 5 months).

Labour   No.

Postnatally   Yes.

Babies   No.

Eucalyptus *(Eucalyptus globulus)*

Part of plant used   Leaves and twigs of the tree.

Where produced   Although native to Australia the tree now grows elsewhere, such as North Africa, the Mediterranean and California.

Aroma   Distinctive strong smell, probably known to most people as it is widely used in pharmaceutical products 'to help clear a stuffy nose'.

Price band   Cheap.

Main properties and effects   Antiseptic; antibiotic; analgesic; anti-inflammatory; anti-viral; diuretic; stimulating.

Main uses   It is primarily used for its effect on the respiratory tract, to help clear mucus and ease congestion. Correctly diluted it is suitable for all ages.

This oil is very strong, so always use on the skin in a 1 per cent dilution or less. It can be used as an antiseptic wash for cuts and grazes and when well diluted in water, gel or a cream can be applied (with bergamot) to cold sores or spots, particularly if inflamed.

Eucalyptus is cooling to the body, so is helpful during feverish illnesses. Use in a very low dilution in baths for urinary infections, particularly when accompanied by a fever. It can be used either in the bath or as a cool compress to help take the unpleasant itch out of chickenpox spots (please consult your aromatherapist for advice on quantities to suit the age of your child). Used in room sprays or vaporisers, it will help cleanse the air and cut down on airborne bacteria. Ideal for places where bugs lurk – lavatories, doctors' waiting rooms, offices, schools, etc. (mix in equal parts with bergamot and lemon for a more agreeable aroma).

Added to a massage blend with other oils, its warming and anti-inflammatory actions helps ease stiff joints, especially in rheumatism and aching muscles.

Ways to use   Body massage; local washes; vaporisation; compresses; skin care; baths (very low dilution).
Preconceptual care   No.
Pregnancy   Yes.
Labour   No.
Postnatally   No.
Babies   Yes.

Geranium *(Pelargonium graveolens)*

Part of plant used   Distilled from the whole plant.
Where produced   Grown in several places, the best coming from Reunion Island.
Aroma   Fresh; flowery.
Price band   Middle.
Main properties and effects   Antiseptic; anti-depressant; astringent; diuretic; fortifying; healing; refreshing; toning; uplifting.
Main uses   Geranium is probably one of the most useful oils in aromatherapy, being helpful to many ailments. Its effect on the body is to balance. Postnatally and in general treatments for everyone, its uplifting aroma can cheer and relieve depression and fatigue, whether used in a massage, a bath or a vaporiser. It stimulates the lymphatic system, relieves fluid retention and the congestion in engorged breasts. It is frequently used in cellulite treatments. It has a regulating action on hormonal balance and is often used alone or in a blend to relieve premenstrual and menopausal symptoms. It is excellent for all types of skin. Used in facial oils, lotions and creams, its action helps to balance the production of sebum (natural oil) in the skin. Blended into a carrier oil and used after a bath or shower, it leaves a delightful fragrance on the skin. Used in compresses, local washes and creams it can help heal wounds and sores.

It can be stimulating, so is best avoided in a massage towards the end of the day. Conversely it makes a good reviving bath oil to use before going out for the evening. Its scent is liked by most people. It blends well with most oils, but is quite powerful and will tend to dominate other oils, so if blending use in moderation. It makes a good oil to spray around the house to freshen up rooms, particularly in old houses, and is useful as an insect repellent.
Ways to use   Face and body massage; facial oil; skin care; baths; showers; local application; compresses; vaporisation.
Preconceptual care   Yes.

Pregnancy   Yes (in low dilution for refreshing rooms and after 5 months for local applications (e.g. oils and gels for fluid retention, etc.))
Labour   Yes.
Postnatally   Yes.
Babies   No.

Jasmine *(Jasminum officinale)*

Part of plant used   Flowers.
Where produced   Egypt; Morocco; India.
Aroma   Highly fragrant and sweet.
Price band   Very expensive.
Main properties and effects   Anti-depressant; antiseptic; anti-spasmodic; aphrodisiac; helpful during labour; increases breast-milk flow; general tonic.
Main uses   With its heavenly fragrance, it is much loved by the perfume industry. For something so delicate, jasmine oil is very strong and only a few drops are needed either when used alone or in a blend. It has an uplifting, calming and boosting effect on the emotions and makes an ideal choice to add to a postnatal massage blend, as it also helps to increase breast-milk flow. During labour it will help to boost confidence, relieve pain and help expel the placenta. Its effects are beneficial for painful periods and helpful for the emotional symptoms sometimes experienced during the menopause. Reputedly an aphrodisiac, its use is strongly indicated in preconceptual care or for emotionally related sexual problems. Added to a cream or used in a facial massage oil, jasmine is very good for dry and sensitive skins.
Ways to use   Body and face massage; baths; showers; vaporisation; skin care.
Preconceptual care   Yes.
Pregnancy   No.
Labour   Yes.
Postnatally   Yes.
Babies   No.

Lavender *(Lavandula officinalis)*

Part of plant used   Distilled from the flower heads.
Where produced   All over Europe.
Aroma   Fresh and floral.
Price band   Cheap.

Main properties and effects   Antiseptic; antibiotic; analgesic; anti-depressant; diuretic; anti-viral; anti-fungal; anti-spasmodic; healing; sedating; toning.

Main uses   This gentle essential oil must rate as one of the most used by aromatherapists. It enhances the other oils it is blended with and mixes well with the majority of oils. Among a wide range of properties, its main effect on the body is to 'normalise' it. Its antiseptic and healing properties help with cuts, wounds, dermatitis, eczema, nappy rash, spots and burns. As with tea-tree oil, it may be used neat in tiny quantities directly on the skin. One of the most important oils in skin care, it helps to encourage cell renewal and minimise scars. Use in a facial oil for any skin type.

It will help regulate menstruation if the body is out of balance. It is used to treat all muscular aches and pains, particularly sharp acute pain. It is recommended for use in labour. Physically and mentally, it makes a relaxing bath oil for anyone. It can help relieve fluid retention and ease aching legs and feet. Use in a massage or compress to relieve headaches and migraine. Its gentle but effective sedative action encourages restful sleep in the young and elderly. In infantile colic it will help calm and relieve pain. Use to treat thrush and athlete's foot in local washes, creams and gels.

Ways to use   Body and face massage; local washes; baths; showers; vaporisation; skin care.

Preconceptual care   No.
Pregnancy   Yes.
Labour   Yes.
Postnatally   Yes.
Babies   Yes.

Lemon *(Citrus limonum)*

Part of plant used   Expressed from the rind.
Where produced   Mainly in the Mediterranean.
Aroma   Fresh and citrus.
Price band   Cheap.
Main properties and effects   Antiseptic; anti-bacterial; anti-fungal; astringent; diuretic; stimulant; tonic.
Main uses   Although the fruit has a sharp acid taste, the oil is known to cut down acidity in the body and is very refreshing. Used widely in beauty care, it is both astringent and healing. Reputedly an age retardant. Add it to face creams and masks to whiten and soften dull dingy skin (neck creams especially). It makes an excellent addition to hand creams. When added to a

mild skin tonic, such as orange flower water, lemon oil will reduce oiliness, freshen greasy skin and tone open pores. Use after shampooing to rinse greasy hair. Due to its mild bleaching action, lemon oil is a long-time favourite in hair rinses for fair hair.

When added to a bath or massage blend, its toning and invigorating action can stimulate a sluggish circulation and help to reduce fluid retention and cellulite. Keep a lotion containing lemon, geranium and cypress oil in the fridge to help soothe throbbing varicose veins.

Lemon in a vaporiser or room spray can cut down on airborne bacteria and freshen the atmosphere. The fresh aroma can ease the nausea experienced in morning sickness.

A 2 per cent dilution in water can be used to bathe cuts and grazes (if the wound is infected use previously boiled and cooled water). Using the same 2 per cent dilution, soak a cotton-wool pad and hold across the bridge of the nose to help control nosebleeds (pinch the nostrils together to help constrict the capillaries, obviously making sure your patient can breath through the mouth first). Seek medical advice if a nosebleed is severe or if nosebleeds happen frequently.

Lemon oil can be used neat to help remove warts and verrucas (not moles – see your G.P.). Put 1 drop straight on to the wart with a cotton bud or the corner of a tissue, or add to the gauze pad of a plaster before applying. Avoid the surrounding healthy skin and keep the wart (or verruca) covered. This is best done twice a day, but if you are rushed in the mornings, do it faithfully every evening for successful results. The wart will eventually just drop off. It is difficult to forecast how long this will take, but the average time is a month.

Ways to use   Body massage; skin care; baths; showers; local application; vaporisation.
Preconceptual care   No.
Pregnancy   Yes.
Labour   No.
Postnatally   Yes.
Babies   No.

Mandarin *(Citrus nobilis)*
Tangerine *(Citrus reticulata)* has the same therapeutic properties as mandarin

Part of plant used   Expressed from the rind.
Where produced   Mostly USA and South America.

Aroma   Orangey; fresh; mild.
Price band   Inexpensive.
Main properties and effects   Antiseptic; refreshing; tonic; digestive stimulant; mild relaxant.
Main uses   Both mandarin and tangerine oil are very gentle and can be used in massages for both young and old. They are useful for all kinds of stomach upsets (whether caused by food poisoning or feeling nervous) and constipation. During pregnancy and postnatally, these two oils make refreshing, calming and fortifying baths. They are the first choice as ingredients in creams and oils to help keep body skin supple in pregnancy. Mix with geranium for a delicious-smelling body oil or lotion.

Their very gentle diuretic effects make them suitable additions to massage blends and baths to help disperse minor fluid retention. When used in a vaporiser their aroma is pleasant and cheering.
Ways to use   Baths; body massage; showers; skin care; vaporisation.
Preconceptual care   No.
Pregnancy   Yes.
Labour   Yes.
Postnatally   Yes.
Babies   Yes.

Marjoram, Sweet *(Origanum marjorana)*

Part of plant used   Flowering tops and leaves.
Where produced   Europe; the Mediterranean.
Aroma   Sweet; warm; powerful.
Price band   Middle.
Main properties and effects   Analgesic; antiseptic; anti-spasmodic; strong sedative; menstrual stimulant; vasodilator.
Main uses   Do not confuse with Spanish marjoram (*Thymus mastichina*), which although called marjoram is from the much stronger thyme family. Sweet marjoram is a strong oil to be used sparingly. It is warm, comforting, calming and encourages sleep, so is as helpful to the insomniac as it is to those suffering from anxiety, stress and unhappiness, whether deep-rooted or acute. Its properties can help reduce high blood pressure, headaches and migraines. It relieves nagging muscular aches, in particular cramps, arthritic pain and sporting injuries. Use mixed in a blend with camomile or lavender. Never massage acute injuries or inflamed joints until the swelling has subsided. Instead use on a compress to ease swelling and pain.

When massaged gently on the lower abdomen its soothing action can help constipation, colic (adults) and menstrual pain. Described as dulling to sexual desire, it might not be the best oil to massage your lover with, unless he or she is suffering from stress, insomnia or torn knee ligaments.

Ways to use   Body massage; baths; showers; compresses; vaporisation.
Preconceptual care   No.
Pregnancy   No.
Labour   No (although some birth units use marjoram during early labour).
Postnatally   Yes.
Babies   No.

Neroli *(Citrus aurantium)*

Part of plant used   Distilled from the flowers of the bitter orange tree (orange water is produced from the distillation water).
Where produced   Mainly Italy and Tunisia.
Aroma   Warm; floral.
Price band   Very expensive.
Main properties and effects   Antiseptic; anti-depressant; anti-spasmodic; anti-inflammatory; aphrodisiac; ultra-relaxing and calming.
Main uses   It is used by the perfume and cosmetic industry (one of the classic oils used in eau-de-Cologne). With its beautiful aroma and the pleasing sensations it arouses, I call this the 'anti-anxiety oil'. It rates among the best oils for dispelling fear, shock, nervous tension, depression and panic attacks, and will calm and relieve the unwelcome effects that these stresses bring to the body, such as laboured breathing, insomnia, mental fatigue, irritability and stomach upsets.

Its value in therapy as a face and body oil is enormous. Neroli helps to stimulate healthy new skin cells and is widely used by aromatherapists in skin-care creams. A facial massage with this luxurious oil not only treats the skin but relaxes mind, body and soul at the same time. Diluted to 1 per cent, it can be used on very delicate skins and for soothing inflamed areas.

Ways to use   Body and face massage; baths; showers; skin care; vaporisation.
Preconceptual care   Yes.
Pregnancy   Yes.
Labour   Yes.
Babies   Yes.

Petitgrain *(Citrus aurantium)*

Part of plant used   Leaves and twigs of the same bitter orange tree that gives us neroli oil.
Where produced   Italy; Tunisia.
Aroma   Floral; fresh; mild.
Price band   Inexpensive.
Main properties and effects   Antiseptic; anti-depressant; sedative; deodorant; refreshing; tonic.
Main uses   As this oil comes from the same tree as neroli, it is not surprising that it shares the same properties, but to a lesser degree. It is not as sedating or calming and its perfume is lighter and fresher. As it leaves one feeling both relaxed and invigorated, it makes it a good choice for someone wanting a massage with the 'neroli aroma', but who doesn't necessarily need the more powerful therapeutic and calming effects of neroli. As a bath oil it has deodorant and refreshing properties and is liked by both men and women. A rather big plus is that it is so much cheaper than neroli, which means that it is more accessible to most people. It makes a refreshing additive to facial oils, creams and aftershave lotions, particularly for greasy or spotty skins.
Ways to use   Body and face massage; baths; showers; vaporisation; skin care.
Preconceptual care   No.
Pregnancy   Yes.
Labour   No.
Postnatally   Yes.
Babies   No.

Rose *(Rosa damascena* – the best rose oil or *Rosa centifolia* – highly fragrant but therapeutically inferior)

Part of plant used   Distilled from the flower petals.
Where produced   Bulgaria; North Africa; Morocco; France; Turkey.
Aroma   Very fragrant; floral.
Price band   Very expensive.
Main properties and effects   Antiseptic; antibiotic; anti-depressant; anti-inflammatory; aphrodisiac; menstrual stimulant; tonic.
Main uses   Rose is a beautiful and much-loved flower with a feminine fragrance to match. In my treatment rooms, rose oil is chosen by patients purely for its scent. Therapeutically rose is a powerful anti-depressant and is especially useful where there is

grief, sadness, shyness and uncertainty. Its feminine qualities make it a useful oil for all premenstrual, period and menopausal problems. Men, however, are not excluded from benefiting from this wonderful oil, as it is said to increase sperm production. Postnatally it is uplifting and I can think of no nicer present for a new mother than a bunch of roses and an aromatherapy product containing a good rose oil (avoid synthetic rose oil – it smells cheap, is cheap and can give you a headache).

It is highly antiseptic and although its high price totally excludes its use as an everyday family antiseptic, it comes into its own when used in a cream for sore, inflamed skin. As a skin tonic, it is suitable even for babies and makes a wonderfully fragrant additive to a plain moisturising cream. Use for dry, sensitive skin, prone to thread veins.

It has a tonic effect on the digestive system, especially the liver. It is especially useful for digestive complaints that are on-going because of long-term stress. For a deliciously relaxing and indulgent bath, add 3–4 drops to the water before stepping in. Rose-water is collected at the same distillation as rose oil and makes a refreshing and mild skin tonic, particularly suitable for dry and sensitive skins. It is also good for red, inflamed eyes. Apply to cotton-wool pads, place over closed eyes and relax for 10 minutes.

Ways to use   Face and body massage; skin care; vaporisation; baths.
Preconceptual care   Yes.
Pregnancy   No.
Labour   Yes.
Postnatally   Yes.
Babies   Yes.

Rosemary *(Rosmarinus officinalis)*

Part of plant used   Distilled from flower heads and leaves.
Where produced   France; Spain.
Aroma   Strong; clean; herby.
Price band   Cheap.
Main properties and effects   Antiseptic; analgesic; general stimulant; menstrual stimulant; astringent; diuretic; tonic.
Main uses   An invigorating and stimulating oil, it helps get things moving. Due to its effect on the circulation, it is widely used in treatments for fluid retention and cellulite. It helps relieve the congestion around varicose veins. It makes an invigorating massage for those lacking in muscular tone or feeling sluggish –

in mind as well as in body. Its non-sedating, pain-relieving qualities help soothe sporting injuries, especially as its diuretic action helps to disperse the fluid that collects around the injury site. Its properties help general aches, pains, and stiffness, whether brought on by activities such as gardening or as the result of joint or rheumatic conditions. As a general tonic, it helps banish feelings of fatigue and is helpful during convalescence. Combined with geranium it makes a good 'after work' or 'early morning' reviving bath or shower. It makes a good postnatal bath oil (as it is stimulating do not use at the end of the day or the effects of the oil may keep you awake).

Rosemary is legendary for its ability to help stimulate the memory and allow for clear thought. In massages and compresses, it can help headaches and migraines and clear a stuffy head.

As a hair tonic, rosemary can help treat dandruff and encourage hair growth. Just as camomile is traditionally used in hair rinses for blond hair, so rosemary is used for dark hair.

Ways to use   Body massage; inhalations; vaporisation; compresses; baths and showers.
Preconceptual care   No.
Pregnancy   No.
Labour   No.
Postnatally   Yes.
Babies   No.

Sandalwood *(Santalum album)*

Part of plant used   Wood chippings from the tree.
Where produced   East India.
Aroma   Warm; exotic; woody.
Price band   Middle.
Main properties and effects   Antiseptic; anti-inflammatory; anti-depressant; aphrodisiac; anti-spasmodic; sedating.
Main uses   For thousands of years sandalwood has been used in traditional Indian medicine and religious ceremonies. It is a very healing and soothing oil, both mentally and physically. It is both a strong urinary and pulmonary antiseptic and has the ability to clear the body of mucus. It can soothe and treat dry coughs, catarrh and sore throats, and ease urinary tract infections. In pregnancy and postnatally, use in a warm bath or a lower abdominal massage to help cystitis. It has a calming action on the digestive system and can help flatulence, diarrhoea, heartburn, colic and nausea.

With its soothing actions, sandalwood is particularly suited to dry, inflamed or allergic skin, but because of its antiseptic and astringent properties, it is also helpful for acne and oily patches. It makes an excellent facial oil blended with jojoba and if you like its rather pronounced smell it makes a nourishing additive to a moisturising cream.

As an anti-depressant and relaxant, sandalwood is an oil to choose where stressful problems have led to a lack of direction or emotional and sexual dullness.

Ways to use   Face and body massage; skin care; baths; showers; vaporisation.
Preconceptual care   Yes.
Pregnancy   Yes.
Labour   No.
Postnatally   No.
Babies   No.

Tea-Tree *(Melaleuca alternifolia)*

Part of plant used   Distilled from the leaves of the tree.
Where produced   Australia.
Aroma   Strong; medicinal.
Price band   Cheap.
Main properties and effects   Antibiotic; antiseptic; anti-fungal; anti-viral; disinfectant.
Main uses   The highly antiseptic powers of tea-tree oil have been known to the Australian Aborigines for thousands of years. It would appear to be a panacea for many infections. Research has shown it to be more powerful than many household disinfectants and antiseptics. It can be used to treat skin and scalp infections, septic cuts, boils and wounds, as well as warts and veruccas. Australian dermatologists have proved it to be more effective at controlling acne than many other skin preparations.

As an anti-fungal agent it is proving to be highly successful at treating conditions such as thrush and athlete's foot.

In tiny amounts is may be used neat on grazes, minor burns, spots and small wounds (be careful with sensitive skins).

It can encourage a quick recovery from viruses and bacterial infections, as it appears to be able to boost the body's immune system.

Ways to use   Baths; body massage; local washes; inhalations; vaporisation; compresses; skin care.
Preconceptual care   No.
Pregnancy   Yes.

Labour   No.
Postnatally   No.
Babies   Yes.

Ylang-ylang *(Cananga odorata)*

Part of plant used   Distilled from flowers from the tree.
Where produced   Java; Madagascar.
Aroma   Sweet; strong; fragrant.
Price band   Cheap to middle.
Main properties and effects   Antiseptic; anti-depressant; aphrodisiac; lowers blood pressure; sedative.
Main uses   It is used on its own or in blends to help calm the acute or long-term physical symptoms that arise from anxiety, nervous tension, fear, shock, anger and emotional problems. It helps to normalise a racing heartbeat and rapid breathing, both experienced when one is frightened and under stress. It helps to lower blood pressure.

Its anti-depressant, relaxant and aphrodisiac properties work well together, particularly on someone who is overworked, tired and under stress. Its exotic perfume adds a lingering fragrance to body lotions, creams and bath oils. Added to facial oils and creams, it is balancing and can be used for all skin types. I find it ideally suited to oily and combination skins.

Ways to use   Face and body massage; baths; showers; skin care.
Preconceptual care   Yes.
Pregnancy   Yes.
Labour   Yes.
Postnatally   Yes.
Babies   No.

Using percentages when making up oils and creams

During pregnancy, it is advisable to use a very low concentration of essential oil when making up massage oils, creams and lotions. Baths and footbaths are not so critical, because in these you usually use a set number of drops in a large volume of water. Dilutions can be worked out to adapt to whatever size bottles or containers you have at home by using percentages.

Percentages for non-pregnant women *(over 16)*

Most aromatherapy massage oils for non-pregnant women are made up to a $2^{1}/_{2}$ per cent concentration (i.e. $2^{1}/_{2}$ per cent of the total volume of massage oil should be made up of essential oils). All you have to do is know how much your container holds in millilitres. Fill this with a carrier oil. Then add half the number of drops of essential oil as there are millilitres of carrier oil. For example:

To a 100 ml bottle of carrier oil add 50 drops of essential oil.
To a 50 ml bottle of carrier oil add 25 drops of essential oil.
To a 10 ml bottle of carrier oil add 5 drops of essential oil.

Percentages for pregnancy

During pregnancy and the postnatal period – and for those with sensitive skins – I suggest you use massage oils with a 1 per cent concentration of essential oil. This means adding approximately half the number of drops of essential oil that you did for the $2^{1}/_{2}$ per cent concentration above. For example:

To a 100 ml bottle of carrier oil add 25 drops of essential oil.
To a 50 ml bottle of carrier oil add 12 drops of essential oil.
To a 12 ml bottle of carrier oil add 3 drops of essential oil.
To a 10 ml bottle of carrier oil add 2 drops of essential oil.

Glossary
of medical terms

Analgesic   Pain-relieving.
Antibiotic   Kills pathogenic bacteria.
Anti-depressant   Mood elevator.
Anti-fungal   Stops growth of mould or fungi.
Anti-inflammatory   Reduces or prevents inflammation.
Antiseptic   Wound-cleaning; prevents microbe development.
Anti-spasmodic   Relieves smooth muscle spasm.
Anti-viral   Destroys certain viruses.
Aphrodisiac   Substance that stimulates sexual desire.
Astringent   Contracts blood vessels and body tissue.
Bacteriocide   Substance that inhibits growth of bacteria.
Balancing   Maintains or returns to a state of equilibrium.
Decongestant   Substance that reduces congestion.
Diuretic   Substance which aids production of urine.
Emmenagogue   Substance that induces menstruation.
Engorged   Congested.
Expectorant   Substance that encourages coughing-up of mucus.
Sedative   Substance that lessens excitement or functional activity.

Addresses

Allison England Aromatherapy Products

I can supply all essential oils mentioned in this book, plus carrier oils and glass bottles. I also have a full range of ready-prepared creams, massage oils and gels to treat a wide variety of complaints, including a full range of skin-care creams. These are available by mail order from:

Allison England Aromatherapy,
The Trees,
97 Main Street,
Little Downham, Ely,
Cambridgeshire CB6 2SX
Telephone and fax: 01353 699236
e-mail: Allison England@dial.pipex.com.
Allison England products are available on the www
http://www.allison.england.dial.pipex.com

Please write enclosing an S.A.E. for a current brochure/price list.

Allison England Retail Products
Pure essential oils
Pure essential oil synergie mixes
Massage and body oils
Aromatic gels
Bath products
Hypo-allergenic skin care
Gift packs

Special Products for Pregnancy,
Labour, New Mothers and Babies
Anti-Stretch Mark Gel/Cream
Anti-Stretch Mark Oil
Pregnancy Relaxing Bath Oil
Labour Day Massage Oil
After-Delivery Healing Bath
    Drops
Aroma Baby Products
Pregnancy Bath/Shower Gel
Camomile and Rose Baby Oil
Camomile and Rose Baby Bath

How to find an aromatherapist
To find an aromatherapist in your area who is qualified in pregnancy massage contact:

The International Federation of Aromatherapists,
Stamford House,
3–5 Chiswick High Road,
London W4 1TH
Telephone: 0181 742 2605

Write enclosing an S.A.E.

Breast-feeding problems
La Leche League,
BM 3424,
London WC1N 3XY
Telephone: 0171 242 1278

La Leche League offers mother-to-mother support for women who want to breast-feed or who have problems with it, trained counsellors on hand. They also offer an electric breast-pump hire service. They have offices in 22 countries and all 50 US states. Find on www under La Leche League.

The National Childbirth Trust (NCT),
Alexandra House, Oldham Terrace,
London W3 6NH
Telephone: 0181 992 8637
lines open 9.30 am–4.30 pm
Fax: 0181 992 5929
Web site www.nctms.co.uk

Write enclosing an S.A.E.

The NCT offers support both during pregnancy and postnatally. Organises local antenatal classes and offers postnatal support by putting new mothers in touch with each other and giving advice on crèche groups. Offers help on breast-feeding, and can supply electric breast pumps for hire.

Preconceptual care
Foresight,
The Association for the Promotion of Preconceptual Care,
28 The Paddock,
Godalming, Surrey GU7 1XD
Telephone: 01483 427 839
Fax: 01483 427 668

Postnatal problems
The Association of Postnatal Illness,
25 Jerden Place,
Fulham,
London SW6 1BE
Telephone: 0171 386 0868
Fax: 0171 386 8885

If you are suffering from postnatal depression or illness, they can put you in touch with someone who has been through a similar experience.

Multiple births
The Administrators,
The Twins and Multiple Births Association (TAMBA),
P.O. Box 30,
Little Sutton,
South Wirral L66 1TH
Telephone: 0151 348 0020

They can offer support and encouragement to parents.

Index

Bold page numbers refer to main entries

air purification/scenting 26–7,76
allergies 28, 38
allergic skin 100
Aloe vera 34
ancient Egypt 15
Angelica 37
aniseed 37
apricot kernel 35
Arabia 17
armoise 38
Arnica 38
aromatherapy
    benefits of in pregnancy 1–7
    definition of 8
    essential oils to avoid 36–8
    pregnancy success stories 3–7
aromatic baths *see* baths
asthma 38
Avicenna 15
avocado 33

baby massage 106–10
    belly 115
    method 108–10
    oils 106–7, 113, 114
    pre-birth 49
    tips 107–8
baby problems 111–21
    colic 107, 114–18
    cradle cap 113
    nappy rash 119–20
    snuffles 111
backache 50–1
baldo leaf 38
base oils 35–6
basil 37
baths
    anti-cellulite 97
    aromatic, generally 23–4
    bidets 23

children's 23–4
footbaths 24
labour 72
nappy rash 120
sitz 23
for toddlers 122
belly massage 115
benzoin **127–8**
bergamot **128**
bidets 23
bitter almond 38
body creams 93
body scrubs 94–5
breasts
    breast-feeding 86–9
    engorgement 88
    massage 61, 87
    mastitis 89
    sore 61
    sore nipples 88–9

Caesarean delivery 80
calamus 38
Calendula 34
camomile
    German **129**
    Roman 117, **129**
camphor 37
carrier oils 33–6
    mixing 35–6
cedarwood 37
cellulite
    anti-cellulite bath 97
    anti-cellulite massage oil 97
    getting rid of 95–7
    and skin brushing 96–7
Chamberland, Dr 18
children's baths 23–4
cinnamon 37
clary sage 37, 69, **129–30**

Cleopatra 16
clove 37
colic 107, 114–8
compresses 24–5
compulsory bed rest 51
conception
    bath mixes for 126
    essential oils to aid 125–6
    failure to conceive 125–6
    massage oils to aid 126
    preconceptual care 124–6
cradle cap 113
cramps 51–2
creams
    body 93
    face 101–3
    percentages when making 142–3
    for thrush 65
Culpepper, Nicholas 17
cypress 31, **130–1**
cystitis 52–3

delivery room
    oils for 76
    perfuming 76
dermatitis 28, 38
diet
    and fluid retention 54
    postnatal 91–2
    and postnatal hair 104–5
    preconceptual 124
    and thrush 64
Dioscoridese 16

eczema 28, 38, 114
emmenagogic oils 36–7
enfleurage 9
epilepsy 38
episiotomy 79
ergomatrine 19
essential oils *see also* oils; massage
    oils; pregnancy, essential
    oils
    absorption of 13–14, 49
    base oils, mixing with 35–6
    Bible references to 15–16
    buying 38–9
    care in use 28, 36–8, 123
    conception, as aid to 125–6
    cost of 9, 38, 39
    definition of 8
    delivery room 76
    extraction of 8–9

guide to 29–38
handling 40–1
history of 15–19
    in childbirth 19–20
in hospitals, use of 20
labour and birth 68–71, 76
labour bath mix 72
methods of use 21–8
patch testing 28
properties and uses 10–11
reference guide to 127–143
safety 36–8
storage 39–40
thrush mix 64
Eucalyptus **131–2**
'evening crying' 114
exercise, postnatal 91–2, 95
expression 9

face
    creams 101–3
    oils 61, 100–1
    scrubs 103
    skin types 99–100
failure to conceive 125–6
faintness 54
fatigue 53–4, 82–4
feet
    and fluid retention 48, 54–5
    footbaths 24
    leg and foot oil 55
    massage 21–2, 48–9
fennel 37
figure recovery 90–2
fluid retention 48, 54–5

Galen 16
Gattefosse, René 18
geranium 32, 70–1, 125, **132–3**
Gerard, John 18
German camomile **129**
Gordon, Yehudi 106
grapeseed 33
Greek physicians 16
groin ache 50–1
gums, sore or bleeding 62

haemorrhoids 55–6
hair
    and diet 104
    fragrant brushing 105
    postnatal 104–5
    pre-wash conditioners 104

rinses 105
shampoo 105
heartburn 56–7
Hinchingbrooke Hospital,
    Huntingdon 20
Hippocrates 16
horseradish 38
hospitals 20
hyssop 37

indigestion 56–7
infantile colic 107, 114–8
inhalations 25
insomnia 57

jaborandi leaf 38
jasmine 37, 70, **133**
jojoba 34
juniper 37

labour
    baths 72
    and birth, generally 68–78
    compress 73
    essential oils for 68–71
    massage 73–5
    massage oil 75
    preparing oils for 71
Lamaze, Fernand 20
Larson, Dr Jan-Helge 115
lavender 29–30, 70, **133–4**
legs
    and cramp 51–2
    and fluid retention 48–9, 54–5
leg and foot oil 55
    massage 48–9, 55
    varicose veins 66–7
lemon 32, **134–5**
lovage 37

mandarin 30, **135–6**
marjoram 37
    Spanish 37, 136
    sweet 37, **136–7**
massage 2, 21–2
    baby 106–10
    baby's pre-birth 49
    base oil for 35–6
    belly 115
    body 21
    breast 61, 87
    facial 22, 61
    foot 21–2, 48–9, 55

labour 73–5
legs 48–9, 55
lotion, varicose vein 67
oils see also essential oils; oils (head-
    ing); pregnancy, essential oils
    anti-cellulite 97
    anti-stretch mark 62–3, 90, 99
    baby 106–7, 113, 114
    cramp 51–2
    facial 61, 100–1
    indigestion 56–7
    labour 75
    legs and feet 55
    preconceptual 126
    standard pregnancy 47, 62
    teething 121
postnatal 83–4
pregnancy see pregnancy massage
mastitis 89
Maury, Marguerite 19
    *Le Capital 'Jeunesse' (The Secret of Life
        and Youth)* 19
Melissa 37
Middle Ages 17, 19
morning sickness 57–8
motherhood, adjustment to see
    postnatal care
mustard 38
myrrh 37

nappy rash 119–20
neroli 30, 70, **137**
nipples, sore 88–9
nose stuffiness 58–9
nosebleeds 58–9
    compress for 59

oils see also essential oils; massage, oils;
        pregnancy, essential oils
    anti-cellulite massage oil 97
    anti-stretch mark 62–3, 90, 99
    baby massage 106–7, 113, 114
    base 35–6
    carrier 33–6
    delivery room 76
    emmenagogic 36–7
    facial 61, 100–1
    percentages when making 142–3
    postnatal 93–4
    postnatal massage 83–4
    preparation of, for labour 71
    Roman camomile baby 117
    teething 121

Olive 35
Origanum 37

palpitations 59–60
Parkinson, John 17
parsley 37
pennyroyal 38
peppermint 37
perineum
  healing 79
  postnatal perineal pain 23
  preparation of 60
petitgrain 30, **138**
pheromones 11–12
postnatal
  blues 80–2
  bodyscrubs 94–5
  care 79–85
  depression 84–5
  diet 91–2
  exercise 91–2, 95
  fatigue 82–4
  hair 104–5
  massage 83–4
  oils 93–4
  perineal pain 23
  recovery 90–97
  skin 98–104
  skin brushing 96–7
pre-birth massage 49
preconceptual care 124–6
pregnancy
  aromatherapy, benefits of, generally
    1–7
  essential oils *see also* essential oils
    (heading)
    to avoid during 36–8
    of greatest use 29–31
    of limited use 31–2
  massage 42–9
    baby's pre-birth 49
    back and shoulder 47
    base oil, recipe for 35–6
    body 47–8
    at home 44–9
    leg and foot 21–2, 48–9, 55
    oil recipe for 47
    professional 42–4
  percentages when making oils
    for 142–3
  use of tampons during 65

Read, Dr Dick Grantly 20
Roman camomile 117, **129**
Romans 16–17
rose 69, 125, **138–9**
rosemary 37, **139–40**
rue 38

sage 37
St John's and St Elizabeth's Hospital,
    London 20
sandalwood 32, 125, **140–1**
sassafras 38
savin 38
savory 37
showers 24
skin
  brushing 96–7
  cleansing 94–5
  postnatal 98–104
  problems 60–1
  properties of 13–14
  types of 99–100
smell, sense of 11–13
solvent extraction 9
southernwood 38
steam distillation 9
stretch marks 62–3
  anti-stretch mark oil 62–3, 90, 99
  standard pregnancy massage oil
    47, 62
sweet almond 33

tampons, use of 65–6
tangerine 31, **135–6**
tansy 38
tarragon 37
tea-tree 32, **141–2**
teething 121
thrush 63–5
Thuja 38
thyme 37
toddler sleeping problems 122–3

Valnet, John 18
  The Practice of Aromatherapy 19
varicose veins 66–7

waist ache 50–1
wheatgerm 34
wintergreen 38
wormwood 38

ylang-ylang 31, 71, 126, **142**

If you have enjoyed

AROMATHERAPY AND MASSAGE FOR MOTHER AND BABY

you may also be interested in the following titles published by Vermilion and Ebury Press:

The National Childbirth Trust Book of Breastfeeding
by Mary Smale   (£7.99)

The National Childbirth Trust Get Into shape After Childbirth
by Gillian Fletcher   (£10.99)

Twins and Multiple Births
by Dr Carol Cooper   (£9.99)

Toddler Taming
by Dr Christopher Green   (£9.99)

The New Baby and Toddler Sleep Programme
by Dr John Pearce   (£7.99)

To obtain your copy, simply telephone the TBS Direct credit-card hotline on 01206 255800.